Principles of Drug Information and Scientific Literature Evaluation

Frank J. Ascione, Pharm.D., Ph.D.
Associate Professor of Pharmacy Administration
University of Michigan, College of Pharmacy
Ann Arbor, Michigan USA

Carol Colvin Manifold, Pharm.D.
Manager, Medical Communications
Immunex Corporation
Seattle, Washington USA

Clinical Assistant Professor
University of Washington School of Pharmacy
Seattle, Washington USA

Mary A. Parenti, Pharm.D.
Chief Executive Officer
Medical Education Systems, Inc.
Philadelphia, Pennsylvania USA

Clinical Assistant Professor of Pharmacy
Philadelphia College of Pharmacy & Science
Philadelphia, Pennsylvania USA

American Pharmaceutical Association, Washington, D.C. USA

Library of Congress Cataloging-in-Publication Data

Ascione, Frank J., 1946-
    Principles of drug information and scientific literature evaluation / Frank J. Ascione, Carol Colvin Manifold, Mary A. Parenti

        p.   cm.

    Includes bibliographical references and index.
    ISBN 0-914768-52-2
    1. Drugs–Information services. 2. Pharmacology–Information services. 3. Pharmacy–Information services. 4. Medical informatics. I. Manifold, Carol Colvin, 1954- . II. Parenti, Mary A., 1962- . III. Title.
    RM301.A75 1994
    025'.6151–dc20   93-41705
                                                        CIP

Printed in the United States of America

Principles of Drug Information and Scientific Literature Evaluation

Frank J. Ascione
Carol Colvin Manifold
Mary A. Parenti

ACKNOWLEDGEMENTS

We gratefully acknowledge the contributions of the following individuals:

Sandra L. Beaird, Pharm.D.
Drug Information Coordinator
Department of Pharmacy
The Jewish Hospital of St. Louis

Ira M. Cohen, Pharm.D.
Chief, Drug Information and
Investigational Drug Service
Department of Pharmacy
University of Michigan Hospitals
Clinical Associate Professor
University of Michigan, College of Pharmacy

Rebecca M.R. Coley, M.S., R.Ph.
Assistant Professor of Pharmacy Administration
Division of Pharmacy Administration
St. Louis College of Pharmacy

Duane M. Kirking, Pharm.D., Ph.D.
Associate Professor of Pharmacy Administration
University of Michigan, College of Pharmacy

Mark C. Pugh, Pharm.D.
Director, Drug Information Service
Medical College of Virginia Hospitals
Clinical Assistant Professor
Department of Pharmacy & Pharmaceutics
Medical College of Virginia
Virginia Commonwealth University

We are grateful to the many publishers and authors who granted us permission to reprint from their publications.

Personal Acknowledgments

To Gloria Francke
We are grateful for your patience and enthusiasm.
--Frank, Carol, and Mary

To Patty, Wendy, and Mark
Thank you for your patience and support. You helped make a difficult task possible.
--Frank

To my many preceptors, colleagues, residents, and students
Thank you for the continual challenges and rewards.
--Carol

To Mom and Dad
Thank you for your love and continuous support throughout my career and during the many
times I challenged you as parents.
--Mary

Preface

An earlier text titled "Principles of Drug Information Services" by Watanabe and Conner[1] served a valuable purpose in providing students and practitioners of drug information with a resource and teaching tool. We are grateful to these authors for publishing the first textbook in this field in 1978.

Since that time, drug information activities have increased in numbers, scope, geography, and impact on patient care. Drug information centers are now located around the world. The impact of drug information may be felt at every level from the individual patient's bedside to the national health care system. As health care resources become more limited, emphasis has increased on the critical analysis of available information regarding possible treatments. We created this new reference book to reflect these and other changes in drug information practice, as well as to provide a more extensive discussion of scientific literature evaluation.

Purpose

The purpose of "Principles of Drug Information and Scientific Literature Evaluation" is to provide a current, comprehensive overview of relevant information and concepts for students and practitioners involved in providing drug information and evaluating scientific literature in the patient care setting.

Organization

The book is organized into four general sections:

I. **Background and Organization**

Section I is intended to be of interest to practitioners who are developing or operating a drug information center. It provides some historical perspective on the development of the drug information specialty, as well as details on the extent to which drug information has evolved, both functionally and geographically. Management topics such as funding and quality assurance are also included.

II.   **Process of Answering Drug Information Questions**

The purpose of Section II is to provide persons who are beginning to learn drug information skills, or who would like to enhance basic skills, with detailed guidance on the "art" as well as "science" of answering drug information questions.

III.   **Scientific Literature Evaluation**

Section III is intended to assist individuals who are interested in obtaining basic skills in scientific literature evaluation, particularly as it applies to clinical drug studies. It provides a stepwise approach to critically evaluating a clinical research article, and includes relevant examples.

IV.   **Appendices**

Numerous appendices are provided in Section IV to supplement the primary material presented in the book.

Target Audience

The orientation of the book is generally toward the health care practitioner, and to students pursuing careers in health care. Although most of the information presented is based on experience in the United States, an attempt has been made to incorporate published information concerning drug information in other countries.

We hope that the book will be helpful for teaching and applying the skills of drug information and scientific literature evaluation.

Frank J. Ascione, Pharm.D., Ph.D.
Carol Colvin Manifold, Pharm.D.
Mary A. Parenti, Pharm.D.

May 1994

Reference

1.   Watanabe AS, Conner CS. Principles of drug information services. Drug Intelligence Publications, Inc., Hamilton, Illinois, 1978.

Contents

SECTION I Background and Organization of Drug Information Services

Chapters 1 through 8 provide practical information on aspects of developing and operating a drug information center. The drug information literature is summarized and organized to serve as a source on the state of drug information practice in the world, particularly in the United States.

Definition

"Drug information," also referred to as "DI," may be defined as the integration of locating, analyzing, applying, and communicating information concerning drugs, usually for use by the person in a decision-making role in patient management. A "drug information service" is a formalized unit with staff and resources dedicated to providing drug information. A "drug information center" is similar to a drug information service, but with the added connotation of a discrete physical setting from which to provide its service.

History of Drug Information Services

The first formalized drug information center was developed in the early 1960s at the University of Kentucky,[1,2] with others following at a number of university medical centers. Several forces contributed to this development. The profession of pharmacy was beginning to focus on a more clinical practice, having greater contact with other health care practitioners, as opposed to a product-oriented practice. The "information explosion" made it difficult for individuals to keep up with the amount of new drug data available. The importance of knowledge concerning drugs (e.g., adverse drug reactions, drug interactions) and its role in patient management was being increasingly recognized. Chapter 3 provides more in-depth discussion of the emergence of the pharmacist as the primary drug information contact among health care or information specialists.

In the late 1960s, drug information centers grew rapidly through funding by the United States National Library of Medicine (NLM) Regional Medical Programs (RMPs) grant for regional or statewide drug information centers.[3-6] The regional drug information centers were located in Connecticut, Florida, Michigan, Nebraska, New Jersey, New Mexico, New York, Ohio, and West Virginia.[6] RMP funding was discontinued in the early 1970s.[4]

In 1968, the American Society of Hospital Pharmacists (ASHP) published a position statement concerning the role of the hospital pharmacist in providing drug information.[7] It lists the following activities a "drug information specialist" should perform:

1. evaluate, select, and utilize drug literature, presenting maximum relevant information with minimum volume, with independent, informed conclusions
2. make full use of institutional and extramural library facilities
3. effectively communicate verbally and in writing
4. contribute to the continuing education of other health professionals
5. directly and indirectly participate in patient care by contributing to the quality of drug usage
6. efficiently utilize electronic data processing methodology for information storage, processing, and retrieval
7. provide professional support to the pharmacy and therapeutics committee.

As the practice of pharmacy evolved and the role of the drug information center became established, this statement was replaced by Standard IV of the ASHP Minimum Standard for Pharmacies in Institutions:[8]

> "The pharmacy is responsible for providing the institution's staff and patients with accurate, comprehensive information about drugs and their use and shall serve as its center for drug information.
>
> - The pharmacist (in cooperation with the organization's librarian, if any) is responsible for maintaining up-to-date drug information resources (both in the pharmacy and at patient-care areas) and using them effectively. The pharmacist, in addition to supplying specific drug information, must be able to furnish objective evaluations of the drug literature and to provide informed opinion on drug-related matters.
> - The pharmacist must keep the institution's staff well informed about the drugs used in the institution and their various dosage forms and packagings. This is accomplished through newsletters, seminars, displays, etc., developed by the pharmacy. No drug shall be administered unless the medical and nursing personnel have received adequate information about, and are familiar with, its therapeutic use, adverse effects, and dosage.
> - The pharmacist must help ensure that all patients are given adequate information about the drugs they receive. This is particularly important for ambulatory, home care, and discharge patients. These patient education activities shall be coordinated with the nursing and medical staffs and patient education department (if any)."

Number, Locations, and Affiliations

Drug information centers are now located in many countries of the world and in several types of professional settings (e.g., hospitals, schools of pharmacy or universities, pharmaceutical associations, pharmaceutical companies).

1. United States

More drug information centers are located in the United States than in any other country.[9] As of 1992, 130 have been reported in the United States and Puerto Rico (Appendix A).[10]

The number and percentage of drug information centers affiliated with a hospital or medical center increased between 1980 and 1986, while the reverse was true between 1986 and 1990 (Table 1-1).[9,11] In addition, the number of drug information centers affiliated with poison control centers has decreased steadily since 1980. This trend is unexpected in view of the opinion that the advantages of combining drug and poison information services outweigh the disadvantages (see Chapter 5).[12]

Table 1-1.   Affiliations of Drug Information Centers[a]

Affiliation[b]	Number (%)[c] of Drug Information Centers			
	1976 n=79	1980 n=96	1986 n=127	1990 n=130
Hospital or medical center	65 (82)	78 (81)[d]	120 (94)[d]	107 (82)
College of pharmacy	44 (56)	60 (63)	74 (58)	98 (75)
Poison control center	23 (29)	36 (38)[d]	24 (19)[d]	2 (2)
College of medicine	18 (23)	20 (21)[d]	46 (36)[d]	47 (36)
College of nursing	11 (14)	13 (14)	30 (24)	...[e]
College of dentistry	10 (13)	5 (5)	1 (<1)	...[e]
College of allied health professions	...[e]	...[e]	19 (15)	...[e]
Library	...[e]	...[e]	33 (26)	...[e]

[a]   Adapted with permission from Rosenberg JM, Martino FP, Kirschenbaum HL, Robbins J. Pharmacist-operated drug information centers in the United States -- 1986. *Am J Hosp Pharm* 1987;44:337-44 and Beaird SL, Coley RMR, Crea KA. Current status of drug information centers. *Am J Hosp Pharm* 1992;49:103-6.

[b]   Each center could have multiple affiliations

[c]   Rounded to nearest whole number

[d]   Significantly different (p <0.05) according to Fisher's exact test

[e]   Data not collected

Many pharmaceutical companies also have drug information centers, or at least staff designated to answer drug information questions from health care professionals. These services can best be located in the *Physicians' Desk Reference* (PDR) manufacturers' index, which lists the telephone number specifically for product or medical information.[13] Pharmaceutical companies may limit the drug information services they provide to consumers, in order to avoid compromising the relationship between the patient and the patient's primary health care professional as well as to minimize liability exposure.

2.   Other Countries

Drug information centers have been established in Canada (Appendix B),[14] Australia, Japan, the Middle East, Nigeria, South Africa, Zimbabwe, Sri Lanka, India,[15] New Zealand, South America, and many European countries.[16-18]

Maguire and D'Arcy surveyed drug information centers in Europe, finding 29 centers in 14 countries (Appendix C).[17] Of these centers, 10 (35%) were hospital-based, 6 (21%) were in pharmaceutical companies, 4 (13%) were provided by pharmaceutical associations, 2 (7%) were in schools of pharmacy or universities, and 7 (24%) fell into an "other" category.

A national Medicines Resource Centre (MeReC) was established in the United Kingdom in December 1989, to interact with the present National Drug Information Network of regional drug information centers. The MeReC does not answer individual drug information questions, but provides "an independent source of drug and prescribing information".[19]

References

1. Amerson AB, Wallingford DM. Twenty years' experience with drug information centers. *Am J Hosp Pharm* 1983;40:1172-8.
2. Parker PF. The University of Kentucky drug information center. *Am J Hosp Pharm* 1965;22:42-7.
3. Evens RP. The state of the art, and future directions, of drug information centers. *Pharm Int* 1985;19:74-7.
4. Groth PE. Regional drug information service benefits: free versus fee-for-service. *Am J Hosp Pharm* 1975;32:26-30.
5. Pearson RE, Salter FJ, Bohl JC, Thudium VF, Phillips GL. Michigan regional drug information network. Part I. Concepts. *Am J Hosp Pharm* 1970;27:911-3.
6. Schweigert BF. Drug information services on a subscription basis. *Am J Hosp Pharm* 1976;33:823-7.
7. Anon. The hospital pharmacist and drug information services. *Am J Hosp Pharm* 1968;25:381-2.
8. ASHP guidelines: minimum standard for pharmacies in institutions. *Am J Hosp Pharm* 1985;42:372-5.
9. Rosenberg JM, Martino FP, Kirschenbaum HL, Robbins J. Pharmacist-operated drug information centers in the United States -- 1986. *Am J Hosp Pharm* 1987;44:337-44.
10. Beaird SL, Coley RMR. 1991/1992 Directory of drug information centers. St. Louis Drug Information Center, St. Louis College of Pharmacy 1992:1-12.
11. Beaird SL, Coley RMR, Crea KA. Current status of drug information centers. *Am J Hosp Pharm* 1992;49:103-6.
12. Troutman WG, Wanke LA. Advantages and disadvantages of combining poison control and drug information centers. *Am J Hosp Pharm* 1983;40:1219-22.
13. *Physicians' Desk Reference*. Medical Economics Publishing, Oradell, NJ, 1993.
14. Anon. Canadian drug information centres. *Can J Hosp Pharm* 1988;41:284-5.
15. Bajaj A, Peswani K. Drug information systems and centres. *Pharm Times* 1988;20:11-3.
16. Gallo GR, Wertheimer AI. An international survey of drug information centers. *Drug Inf J* 1985;19:57-61.
17. Maguire ME, D'Arcy PF. Present drug information services in Europe including 'The two pharmacists of Verona'. *Int Pharm J* 1990;4:49-56.
18. Smith JM. Drug information services -- an update. *Int Pharm Rev* 1988;1:1-4.
19. Anon. *Scrip* 1990; No. 1518/9:9.

Need for Drug Information Services

Drug information services generally meet two basic needs in organized health care settings:

1. *Patient-Specific Clinical Information*

   The drug information center serves as a central site for storage and retrieval of drug information, as well as providing specially trained staff to respond to patient-specific inquiries involving drug therapy.

2. *Institutional Drug Use Overview*

   The drug information center is often responsible for programs geared toward ensuring appropriate, cost-effective drug use throughout the institution. Activities usually include coordination of pharmacy and therapeutics committees, management of the hospital or managed care corporate formulary, publishing newsletters, drug utilization evaluation, and providing inservice education to professional staff (see "Functions" below).

A third need, filled by drug information centers which answer calls from consumers is to provide information to consumers who may not have obtained sufficient information from their primary health care provider. Golightly and colleagues queried 1522 patients concerning the reason they contacted the drug information center: 822 (54%) did so "because their physician or pharmacist had failed to provide any information about the uses and effects of prescribed medications"; 332 (22%) "considered the information provided by the physician or pharmacist to be unclear or in some way inadequate"; and 368 (24%) wanted "to verify the accuracy of information provided by the physician or pharmacist".[1]

Functions of Drug Information Services

1. *Responding to Drug Information Questions*

   a. Types and numbers of questions

   The types of questions received by drug information centers and their incidence, as surveyed by Rosenberg and colleagues on three occasions in a ten-year period, are listed in Table 2-1.[2] The number of questions received monthly by these drug information centers and those surveyed by others in 1990 varied from less than 50 to more than 200 (Table 2-2).[2-3] The volume of inquiries is not a sufficient measure of workload, as the complexity of the inquiries varies widely. "Judgmental" responses (those requiring evaluation of options or synthesis of data) were required for an average of 46% (range 0 to 90%) of the drug information requests, as reported by the drug information centers responding to the 1986 survey.[2] Dombrowski and Visconti found the mean number of questions in drug information centers not affiliated with a poison control center to be 212 per month; drug information centers associated with a poison control center reported a monthly average of 264 questions, of which 40% were poison-related.[4] Responding to drug information questions typically requires one-third to one-half of staff time.[2,4]

Table 2-1.   Types of Questions Received by Drug Information Centers[a]

Request Category	%[b] of All Requests		
	1976 (n=74)	1980 (n=75)	1986 (n=115)
Therapeutic use	13	14	16
Dosage	16	11	11
Identification of an American product	12	9	9
Adverse reactions	9	8	8
Availability	8	8	8
Side effects	7	9	9
Identification of foreign product	3	7	6
Pharmaceutical compatibility	6	6	...[c]
Toxicity	8	6	5
Interactions	4	6	7
Therapeutic compatibility	4	4	...[c]
Metabolism	2	3	...[c]
Contraindications	2	3	2
Therapeutic drug monitoring	...[c]	...[c]	4
Pharmacokinetic calculations	...[c]	...[c]	5
Other	8	7	10

[a]   Adapted with permission from Rosenberg JM, Martino FP, Kirschenbaum HL, Robbins J. Pharmacist-operated drug information centers in the United States -- 1986. *Am J Hosp Pharm* 1987;44:337-44.

[b]   Rounded to nearest whole number

[c]   Data not collected

Table 2-2.   Number of Questions Received per Month by Drug Information Centers[a]

Number of Questions	Number (%)[b] of Drug Information Centers			
	1976 (n=68)	1980 (n=83)	1986 (n=112)	1990 (n=125)
≤ 50	9 (13)	20 (24)	21 (19)	20 (16)
50-100	18 (26)	10 (12)	24 (21)	32 (26)
101-150	13 (19)	14 (17)	20 (18)	16 (13)
151-200	7 (10)	13 (16)	13 (12)	19 (15)
>200	21 (31)	26 (31)	34 (30)	38 (30)

[a]   Adapted with permission from Rosenberg JM, Martino FP, Kirschenbaum HL, Robbins J. Pharmacist-operated drug information centers in the United States -- 1986. *Am J Hosp Pharm* 1987;44:337-44 and Beaird SL, Coley RMR, Crea KA. Current status of drug information centers. *Am J Hosp Pharm* 1992;49:103-6.

[b]   Rounded to nearest whole number

In their European survey, Maguire and D'Arcy reported the volume of drug information requests in a different manner: the number of drug information centers receiving a number of questions within a specified range (Table 2-3).[5] The mean number of questions received by these centers was 4,313 per year (lower limit not specified, upper limit 35,000; Table 2-4). Many centers reported a very high (>80%) percentage of "Drug Use" inquiries, with "Drug Abuse" and "Poisons" questions contributing less than 15% (with the exception of the center in Nijmegen, The Netherlands, for which 40% of calls involved "Drug Abuse").

Table 2-3.   Number of Questions Received by the Drug Information Centers[a]

Number of Questions per Year	Number (%) of Drug Information Centers Involved
35,000	1 (3%)
10,000-20,000	4 (14%)
2,000-6,000	7 (24%)
1,000-1,400	5 (17%)
1,000	6 (21%)
not available	6 (21%)

[a]   Adapted with permission from Maguire ME, D'Arcy PF. Present drug information services in Europe including 'The two pharmacists of Verona'. *Int Pharm J* 1990;4:49-56.

Table 2-4. Drug Information Services -- Inquiry Category[a]

Center	Total	Number				Percentage			
		DU	DA	PS	O	DU	DA	PS	O
Vienna	13000	12350	650	N	N	95	5	N	N
Brussels (1)	14600	NA	NA	NA	NA	NA	NA	NA	NA
Brussels (2)	3422	3422	N	N	N	100	N	N	N
Copenhagen	15000	7500	750	300	6450	50	5	2	43
Paris	10000	9500	N	500	N	95	N	5	N
Frankfurt	20000	19000	1000	N	N	95	5	N	N
Dublin (1)	NA	NA	NA	NA	NA	NA	NA	NA	NA
Dublin (2)	69	54	8	N	7	78	12	N	10
Dublin (3)	NA	NA	NA	NA	NA	NA	NA	NA	NA
Dublin (4)	97	96	N	1	N	99	N	1	N
Dublin (5)	1293	1267	N	26	N	98	N	2	N
Dublin (6)	NA	NA	NA	NA	NA	NA	NA	NA	NA
Milan (1)	NA	NA	NA	NA	NA	NA	NA	NA	NA
Milan (2)	NA	NA	NA	NA	NA	NA	NA	NA	NA
Milan (3)	277	277	N	N	N	100	N	N	N
Torino (4)	NA	NA	NA	NA	NA	NA	NA	NA	NA
Verona (5)	600	402	54	18	126	67	9	3	21
The Hague (1)	5372	NA	NA	NA	NA	NA	NA	NA	NA
Nijmegen (2)	2500	1375	1000	125	N	55	40	5	N
Oslo	4000	3600	400	N	N	90	10	N	N
Lisbon	3115	NA	NA	NA	NA	NA	NA	NA	NA
Madrid	1594	1274	80	240	N	80	5	15	N
Stockholm	17500	10325	875	525	5775	59	5	3	33
Bern (1)	35000	29750	N	5250	N	85	N	N	15
Lausanne (2)	700	630	35	35	N	90	5	5	N
London[b] (1)	2500	NA	NA	NA	NA	NA	NA	NA	NA
Cardiff (2)	3491	NA	NA	NA	NA	NA	NA	NA	NA
Belfast (3)	1681	NA	NA	NA	NA	NA	NA	NA	NA
Edinburgh (4)	1325	NA	NA	NA	NA	NA	NA	NA	NA
	125078	98422	6852	7446	12358				
Mean	4313 (100%)	3393 (79%)	236 (5%)	257 (6%)	426 (10%)				

[a] Adapted with permission from Table 12 in Maguire ME, D'Arcy PF. Present drug information services in Europe including 'The two pharmacists of Verona'. *Int Pharm J* 1990;4:49-56.

[b] North East Thames

DU = Drug Use   DA = Drug Abuse   PS = Poisons   O = Other   NA = Not available   N = No/Nil

b. Types of requestors

1) consumers

In contrast to poison control centers, which are intended to serve consumers as well as health care professionals, very few drug information centers openly provide information to consumers. A 1987 publication lists 10 drug information centers in the United States which promote themselves as available to consumers.[6] Several of these centers also serve as poison control centers. The AIDS Clinical Trials Information Service (ACTIS) of the U.S. Public Health Service provides current information on government and privately sponsored clinical trials to patients with AIDS and their families (1-800-243-7012 or 1-301-217-0023).[7] A similar function is provided by the National Cancer Institute for cancer patients (1-800-4-CANCER).

A group of pharmacists from the University Hospitals of Cleveland and PIRL Consultants of Cleveland have established a unique forum for dissemination of drug information to consumers through "The Pharmacy", a computerized bulletin board service (BBS) on a local public access BBS, the Cleveland FreeNet.[8] The service is also available to other health care providers and, in addition to providing a community service, enhances the visibility of pharmacists.

Although answering drug information calls from consumers is not a stated objective for most drug information centers, professional staff will generally answer such calls.[6] Reasons cited for not answering questions from consumers generally relate to ethical conflicts (e.g., fatal dose for suicide attempt) or liability issues. Chapter 7 provides further discussion of ethical issues in providing drug information.

An extensive study by Chaplin in the United Kingdom concluded, "there is a demand for drug information for the public and -- providing appropriate discussion and consultation take place -- there is widespread support for this from professional organizations".[6] However, the cost of providing a comprehensive service in the United Kingdom was estimated to be £ 500,000 or approximately $900,000 (bank draft rate January 1992) per year. Chaplin concluded that it is premature to establish a full drug information service to the public (consumers) in the United Kingdom and that a pilot study is needed to determine a public drug information center's true costs and benefits.[6]

2) health care professionals

Based on data from three surveys, equal numbers (approximately one-third each) of inquiries to drug information centers come from physicians and pharmacists,[2-4] with nurses accounting for about 15%.[2-3] Interestingly, centers affiliated with educational institutions receive a higher proportion of calls from pharmacists than physicians; the reverse is true for centers not affiliated with an educational institution.[4] The different proportion of calls is probably due to educational institutions frequently having pharmacists accessible in patient care areas, to whom physicians and other health care professionals turn for drug information. Thus, the number of physicians calling a drug information service directly is reduced. The pharmacists in the patient care areas will call the drug information center if they do not have adequate resources to answer the question.

3) European data

In the surveys conducted by Maguire and D'Arcy in Europe, the drug information centers received an average of 77% of requests from pharmacists, 9% from physicians, 2% from nurses, 3% from the public (consumers), and 9% from others, such as the military and embassies.[5] The range of percentages of requestors in these categories varied widely (Table 2-5).

Table 2-5.   Drug Information Services -- Inquiry Source[a]

| Center | Total | Source | | | | | Percentage | | | | |
		P	Phy	N	Pc	O	P	Phy	N	Pc	O
Vienna	13000	6500	2600	N	2600	1300	50	20	N	20	10
Brussels (1)	14600	13140	292	N	N	1168	90	2	N	N	8
Brussels (2)	3422	2806	240	N	N	376	82	7	N	N	11
Copenhagen	15000	13500	450	300	450	300	90	3	2	3	2
Paris	10000	7300	1900	N	200	600	73	19	N	2	6
Frankfurt	20000	16000	400	400	200	2000	80	2	2	1	15
Dublin (1)	NA	NA	NA	NA	NA	NA	NA	NA	NA	NA	NA
Dublin (2)	69	14	N	N	54	N	20	2	N	78	N
Dublin (3)	NA	NA	NA	NA	NA	NA	NA	NA	NA	NA	NA
Dublin (4)	97	13	64	14	1	5	13	67	14	1	5
Dublin (5)	1293	789	207	103	N	194	61	16	8	N	15
Dublin (6)	NA	NA	NA	NA	NA	NA	NA	NA	NA	NA	NA
Milan (1)	NA	NA	NA	NA	NA	NA	NA	NA	NA	NA	NA
Milan (2)	NA	NA	NA	NA	NA	NA	NA	NA	NA	NA	NA
Milan (3)	277	40	137	1	87	12	14	50	1	31	4
Torino (4)	NA	NA	NA	NA	NA	NA	NA	NA	NA	NA	NA
Verona (5)	600	198	324	66	6	6	33	54	11	1	1
The Hague (1)	NA	NA	NA	NA	NA	NA	NA	NA	NA	NA	NA
Nijmegen (2)	2500	250	750	1000	125	375	10	30	40	5	15
Oslo	4000	1200	2400	160	120	120	30	60	4	3	3
Lisbon	3115	2624	165	N	38	188	84	5	N	5	6
Madrid	1594	1435	63	16	48	32	90	4	1	3	2
Stockholm	17500	15225	175	N	1050	1050	87	1	N	6	6
Bern (1)	35000	29750	700	N	N	4550	85	2	N	N	13
Lausanne (2)	700	91	217	315	7	70	13	31	45	1	10
London[b] (1)	NA	NA	NA	NA	NA	NA	NA	NA	NA	NA	NA
Cardiff (2)	3491	2024	943	244	N	279	58	27	7	N	8
Belfast (3)	1681	841	504	168	N	168	50	30	10	N	10
Edinburgh (4)	1325	570	543	159	N	53	43	41	12	N	4
	149264	114310	13075	2946	5086	13846					
Mean	7108	5443	622	140	242	659					
(%)	(100%)	(77%)	(9%)	(2%)	(3%)	(9%)					

[a]   Adapted with permission from Table 11 in Maguire ME, D'Arcy PF. Present drug information services in Europe including 'The two pharmacists of Verona'. *Int Pharm J* 1990;4:49-56.

[b]   North East Thames

P = Pharmacist Phy = Physician N = Nurse Pc = Public O = Other NA = Not Available N = No/Nil

2. Pharmacy and Therapeutics Committee and Formulary Support

One of the most common ways in which a drug information center can influence drug use in a controlled health care setting (i.e., a hospital or managed health care organization) is by providing objective, complete reviews of drugs for formulary consideration. Surveys have revealed that 69% to 89% of drug information centers provide support of some sort to a Pharmacy and Therapeutics (P & T) Committee.[2-4] In their survey, Dombrowski and Visconti found that 86.7% of the responding drug information centers located in hospitals maintained a formulary of approved drugs.[4]

3. Drug Utilization Review / Drug Utilization Evaluation

"Drug Utilization Review" (DUR) has been defined by Brodie and Smith as "an authorized, structured, and continuing program that reviews, analyzes, and interprets patterns (rates and costs) of drug usage in a given health care delivery system against predetermined standards".[9] In more simplistic terms, DUR is a program to ensure that medication use is safe, rational, and cost-effective. In recent years, the term "Drug Utilization Evaluation" (DUE) has generally replaced DUR in the institutional setting. This term more accurately connotes the step beyond simply collecting data on drug use, but evaluating this information and assessing mechanisms for correcting prescribing problems, if needed.

Between 60% and 70% of hospital drug information centers participate in DUR or DUE activities.[2-4] Staff pharmacists also participate in these programs, particularly in decentralized pharmacies with proximity to patient records.

Future DUE activities will likely incorporate methods for gaining a broader perspective for evaluating the overall management of patients. Measures of clinical outcome and total resource consumption for particular diseases will likely be included.

4. Adverse Drug Reaction (ADR) Reporting

The United States Food and Drug Administration (FDA) requests that ADRs be reported under a Medical Products Reporting Program (MEDWatch) using the FDA form 3500 (Appendix D).[10,11] This form may also be used for reporting product quality problems. Reports may be submitted either directly to the FDA or to the manufacturer, who will forward the report to the FDA. The FDA may be contacted at 1-800-FDA-1088 to obtain copies of the form or instructions for completing it. A major contributor to the FDA's program is the United States Pharmacopeia (USP) Practitioners' Reporting Network (PRN), a national reporting system that enables health care professionals to report concerns of quality, safety, or performance of pharmaceuticals, radiopharmaceuticals, animal drug products, devices, or laboratory products. ADRs should be reported to the USP Drug Product Problem Reporting Program, a division of the USP-PRN, using the Drug Product Problem reporting form (Appendix D). The information received in each USP report is forwarded to the FDA and to the product manufacturer.

In an institutional setting, responsibility for coordinating an ADR reporting program usually is assumed by the pharmacist; when a drug information center is present, this function is usually coordinated by the drug information center. Approximately 50% to 85% of drug information centers participate in ADR reporting programs.[2-4] An example of a drug information center-based ADR reporting program is provided by Michel and Knodel.[12]

5. *Patient Counseling*

Direct-to-patient activities such as patient counseling and admission and discharge interviews are not usually a function of drug information centers; less than 25% of drug information centers participate in these activities.[2]

6. *Newsletters*

In the United States, over 85% of drug information centers prepare and distribute newsletters to hospital staff.[3] The mean frequency of newsletter publication is 9.4 +/- 4.8 times per year.[4] Approximately 50% of all drug information centers send their newsletters to other hospital pharmacies, while about 33% send newsletters to community physicians.[4] Very few drug information centers (5 of 98 responding in the survey by Dombrowski and Visconti) send their newsletters to consumers.[4] According to the survey conducted by Maguire and D'Arcy, 21 (72%) of the 29 European drug information centers produce newsletters (Table 2-6).[5]

Table 2-6.   Drug Information Services - Bulletin Publication[a,b]

Center	Title	Frequency	Circulation
Brussels (1)	New Drugs	Monthly	All Physician Pharmacist (PPD)-Belgium
Brussels (2)	Folia Pharmacotherapeutica	Monthly	All PPD-Belgium
Paris	PCH Informations	10/Year	1300
Frankfurt	Pharmazeutische Zeitung	Weekly	27000
Dublin (1)	Irish Pharmacy Journal	Monthly	2000
Dublin (2)	Counselling Analgesic Service	With sponsorship	250
	Drug Abuse in Ireland	Wide circulation for Health Educ. Bureau	
Dublin (3)	Annual Report	Annually	Physicians (Phy)
	Adverse Reactions	Annually	Pharmacists (P)
	Drug Usage Booklets	Annually	Pharmaceutical Industry
Dublin (5)	Drug Digest	Quarterly	2000 IPS members
Milan (1)	Meeting & Courses	Monthly	180
	Library List	Monthly	120
	Bibliography Survey	Monthly	80
	Alert-Pharmacotherapy Update	Weekly	200
	Reviews in Pharmacobiology	Weekly	200
Milan (3)	Ricerca Protica	Bimonthly	3500
Verona (5)	Bollettino Aggiornamenti	Quarterly	1000
Oslo	Terapi Spalten	12-24/Year	1200 Phy/Hospital P (HP)/Students
Lisbon	Information for CEDIME	Occasionally	2500
	Farmacia Portuguesa	Bimonthly	3200
Madrid	Panorma Actual del Medic.	Monthly	NA
Stockholm	Aktuellt om Lakemedel		
	Actualities about Drugs	Monthly	3000
	Varjehanda om Sortimentet	Quarterly	2000
	Sjukhusfarmaci (Hosp Pharm)	Bimonthly	500
	IA-Kontakt (Contact for Information Pharmacists)	Annually	400
	Information about Newly Registered Drugs	Annually	850
Lausanne	Bulletin d'information pour les Soins Infermaries	Monthly	120
London	Netalert	Weekly	250 HP
	Pharmfax	Bimonthly	250 HP
	Infonet	Bimonthly	3200 Community P (CP)
Cardiff	Phocus	Bimonthly	300 HP
	Drug Information	Bimonthly	1000 CP
	Drug Information	Quarterly	1800 General Practitioners (GP)
Belfast	Journal Title	Weekly	36 HP
	Pharmafax	Monthly	20 HP
	Pharmacy Update	Quarterly	600 HP/CP
	Drug Data	Quarterly	4500 HP/Phy/CP/GP/Others (O)
Edinburgh	Lothian Health Brd Info Rev	Monthly	1500 HP/Phy/GP/Nurses

[a] Adapted with permission from Table 9 in Maguire ME, D'Arcy PF. Present drug information services in Europe including 'The two pharmacists of Verona'. *Int Pharm J* 1990;4:49-56.

[b] Information not available for Vienna, Copenhagen, Dublin (4), Dublin (6), Milan (2), Torino (4), The Hague, Nijmegen), Bern

7. *Continuing Education (CE) Programs*

According to a 1990 survey, 46% of drug information centers serve as a training site for hospital pharmacist staff development,[3] and many are approved providers of pharmaceutical continuing education (CE) by the American Council on Pharmaceutical Education (ACPE).[13] Most drug information centers also provide CE programs for other hospital staff. Some prepare CE materials on a contractual basis for other customers.[4]

8. *Investigational Drug Studies*

Involvement of drug information centers in investigational drug studies varies widely. In the survey conducted by Dombrowski and Visconti, 50% of the responding drug information centers maintained files on investigational drugs.[4] Other activities related to investigational drug use were data collection and evaluation, inventory control, protocol set-up, and enrolling patients.

9. *Research*

As many as 50% of drug information centers participate in research activities.[3,4] According to one survey, 31 drug information centers conducted 94 projects in a five-year period.[4] Funding information was provided for 38 of these 94 projects (Table 2-7). Industry funded the largest number of projects, but the government provided the greatest amount of funding. The purpose of most of the research projects was to assess investigational drug therapy, efficacy, and safety. Other projects involved FDA-approved drugs or research related to the administrative aspects of providing drug information services.

Table 2-7.   Source and Amount of Funding for Drug Information Center Research Projects[a]

Source	Total Projects Funded[b]	Total Amount of Funding ($)	Mean Amount of Funding per Project ($)
Industry	21	477,230	22,725
Government	6	784,900	130,817
Hospital	4	6,600	1,650
College	2	22,150	11,075
Private	1	24,000	24,000
Other (combination of sources)	4	263,000	65,750
Summary	38[b]	1,577,880	mean 41,523

[a] Adapted with permission from Dombrowski SR, Visconti JA. National audit of drug information centers. *Am J Hosp Pharm* 1985;42:819-26.

[b] Based on responses of 31 drug information centers

10. *Drug Information Education*

a. Students

In 1986, 75% of 127 drug information centers reported providing training to baccalaureate-level pharmacy students, 48% to Pharm.D. students, and 16% to M.S. pharmacy students. Education was provided to medical students, interns, and residents by 28% of the drug information centers.[2]

Ninety-four percent of colleges of pharmacy responding to a 1984 survey reported some type of formal drug information education in their programs; 49 of these colleges had a drug information center on campus.[14] The educational programs cited were didactic and/or experiential, and varied widely in required hours. Many of the programs were elective rather than mandatory courses. The authors concluded that many pharmacy students were not receiving adequate training in drug information.

Hartzema and colleagues found little published information regarding drug information education in countries other than the United States.[15] They surveyed members of the academic section of the Fédération Internationale Pharmaceutique (FIP) regarding the extent to which drug information education was provided in their curricula, and received responses from 19 countries. Responses varied widely, with the conclusions indicating two primary barriers to further drug information education: 1) availability of faculty and material resources, and 2) lack of time in curricula.

b. Pharmacy residents, drug information residents, and drug information fellows

According to a 1990 survey, 50% of drug information centers provide training to pharmacy residents.[3] Approximately one dozen drug information centers provide advanced or specialized residencies or fellowships in drug information.[16-17] A number of pharmaceutical companies offer one-year specialized residency opportunities in drug information.

The American Society of Hospital Pharmacists (ASHP) has approved and published standards and learning objectives for residency training in drug information practice (Appendix E).[18] This standard supplements the Society's standard for specialized pharmacy residency training programs.[19] At the time this Chapter was written, a new standard was in preparation.

c. Pharmacy staff

An interactive course in drug information skills, which offered 12 hours of continuing education credit, was developed for pharmacy staff at a tertiary care hospital by faculty of a nearby school of pharmacy.[20] Each session, which was offered on two separate days to facilitate attendance, utilized a handbook, wall charts, computer demonstrations, and small group discussion to emphasize information exchange among peers.

11. Drug Product Procurement

To optimize drug therapy and reduce pharmacy costs within the Veterans Affairs (VA) health care system, in addition to patient care responsibilities, the drug information service of the Department of Veterans Affairs (VA) central office in Washington, D.C. is involved in a number of diverse activities, many of which are related to drug product procurement.[21] These include:

  a. making recommendations for contract bidding on therapeutically equivalent products
  b. identifying prescription duplication within the system
  c. reporting product defects
  d. planning drug procurement in unique situations, such as during war
  e. developing gender-specific therapy
  f. evaluating the appropriateness of purchasing only brand name products for certain agents
  g. compiling national drug use data
  h. projecting drug price increases.

References

1. Golightly LK, Davis AG, Budwitz WJ, et al. Documenting the activity and effectiveness of a regional drug information center. *Am J Hosp Pharm* 1988;45:356-61.
2. Rosenberg JM, Martino FP, Kirschenbaum HL, Robbins J. Pharmacist-operated drug information centers in the United States -- 1986. *Am J Hosp Pharm* 1987;44:337-44.
3. Beaird SL, Coley RMR, Crea KA. Current status of drug information centers. *Am J Hosp Pharm* 1992;49:103-6.
4. Dombrowski SR, Visconti JA. National audit of drug information centers. *Am J Hosp Pharm* 1985;42:819-26.
5. Maguire ME, D'Arcy PF. Present drug information services in Europe including 'The two pharmacists of Verona'. *Int Pharm J* 1990;4:49-56.
6. Chaplin S. Implications of the American experience of public drug information for hospital pharmacy. *Proc Guild Hosp Pharm* 1987;24:26-55.
7. Minor JR. How can the latest information on HIV and AIDS clinical trials be obtained? *Am J Hosp Pharm* 1990;47:1129-30.
8. Bednarczyk EM, Kyllonen K, Marcus P, Mendel S. Establishment of a drug information service on a public access computer bulletin board (abstract). *Pharmacotherapy* 1992;12:497.
9. Brodie DC, Smith WE. Constructing a conceptual model of a drug utilization review. *Hospitals* 1976;50:143-9.
10. Kessler DA. Introducing MEDWatch. A new approach to reporting medication and device adverse effects and product problems. *JAMA* 1993;269:2765-8.
11. Department of Health and Human Services, Food and Drug Administration. Form for reporting serious adverse events and product problems with human drug and biological products and devices; availability. *Federal Register* 1993;58(105):31596-610.

12. Michel DJ, Knodel LC. Program coordinated by a drug information service to improve adverse drug reaction reporting in a hospital. *Am J Hosp Pharm* 1986;43:2202-5.
13. Anon. Approved providers of continuing pharmaceutical education. American Council on Pharmaceutical Education, Chicago, Illinois, 1992.
14. Kirschenbaum HL, Rosenberg JM. Educational programs offered by colleges of pharmacy and drug information centers within the United States. *Am J Pharm Ed* 1984;48:155-7.
15. Hartzema AG, Rosenberg L, Temple DJ, Wertheimer AI. Drug information management and provision skills taught to pharmacy students. An international perspective. *J Soc Admin Pharm* 1988;5:59-63.
16. American Society of Hospital Pharmacists Special Interest Group on Drug and Poison Information Practice. Networking Brochure. November 1987.
17. Kirkwood CF. Residency programs in drug information. *Am J Hosp Pharm* 1984;41:14-6.
18. American Society of Hospital Pharmacists. ASHP supplemental standard and learning objectives for residency training in drug information practice. *Am J Hosp Pharm* 1982;39:1970-2.
19. American Society of Hospital Pharmacists. ASHP accreditation standard for specialized pharmacy residency training (with guide to interpretation). *Am J Hosp Pharm* 1980;37:1229-32.
20. Elliott DP, Burke KW, Lorenzo AG, Hess JA. Drug information course for pharmacy staff development. *Am J Hosp Pharm* 1992;49:2935-8.
21. Haynes LM, Patterson AA, Wade SU. Drug information service for drug product procurement in the Veterans Affairs health-care system: preliminary experience. *Am J Hosp Pharm* 1992;49:595-8.

Chapter 3

Role of the Pharmacist and Impact of Drug Information Services

---

Role of the Pharmacist in Drug Information Services

Why is the pharmacist the best person to be responsible for providing drug information? As a group, pharmacists have more extensive education concerning drug therapy compared with other health care professionals. The clinical, administrative, and distributive functions of pharmacists are inseparable, making the pharmacist the logical contact for practical information for patient application. For example, the pharmacist more than any other health care professional is likely to be able to integrate information on efficacy, safety, formulary status, cost, preparation, and delivery of a particular drug therapy.

Ideally, the drug information provider should be knowledgeable about data storage and retrieval methods, be able to objectively evaluate the literature, and have sufficient clinical training to be able to apply the information to the specific patient situation. In addition, the drug information provider should be able to effectively communicate the information to the patient, other health care professionals, or other audiences such as a hospital administrator or the lay press. To quote a British drug information pharmacist, "It is important to distinguish between the role of the medical library and the pro-active, evaluative role that should be the model for drug information. The future of drug information rests on its involvement in, and influence on, therapeutic decisions at the individual or organizational level; passive provision of information in a 'library-mode' is likely to be a diminishing role as the application of information technology to drug data is extended".[1]

This philosophy is consistent with Walton's[2] distinction of two different types of drug information services:

1. the drug literature specialist (drug documentation specialist), whose principal functions are to accumulate, organize, and expedite access to drug literature, and

2. the drug information specialist (clinical drug communication specialist), whose focus is to enhance the clinician's quality of patient care by supplying carefully evaluated, selected literature evidence to justify specific drug usage practices.

Impact of Drug Information Services

Due to the number of factors which influence prescribers' decisions and patient outcomes, it is difficult to determine the extent of impact of any one factor, such as a drug information center. Nevertheless, limited evidence suggests that the effect of drug information services is very positive. Examples of studies undertaken to determine the impact of drug information services are described below:

- Sixty-five percent of drug information centers responding to one survey indicate that the drug information center has had a measurable impact on physicians' prescribing practices; 31% of the centers claim to have demonstrated an impact based on audits of patient charts and follow-up discussions with physicians or patients, among other measures.[5]

- Cardoni and Thompson measured the impact of a drug information service's responses by interviewing requestors after the answer was provided (how long after was not specified).[4] Among a total of 491 requests received during three and one-half months, 443 (90%) were followed up (reasons for lack of follow-up were not given). Of these, 421 (95%) requests were said to be related to patient care. Of the requests related to patient care, 350 (83%) were patient-specific. For the 350 patient-specific requests, the requestors interviewed indicated that the information provided was useful in 329 (94%). An effect on patient outcome was said to have occurred in 202 (58%) of these cases; no effect was reported in 77 (22%), and an indeterminate effect was reported in 71 (20%). For those cases in which patient outcome was affected, 157 (78%) reported a positive effect, while 45 (22%) reported an indeterminate outcome (e.g., insufficient time had passed to see control of chronic disease). Examples of positive effects on patients included promotion of patient well-being through improved nursing care, more knowledgeable monitoring of the patient, financial benefit, or greater understanding of the goals of therapy by the health care team. No difference was seen among physicians, pharmacists, and nurses in the percentage of requests reported to result in positive effects on patients.

  Of the 491 requests received by the drug information center, 11% were considered to be "judgmental" and 89% were considered "nonjudgmental". The authors indicated that a response need not be "judgmental" in order to have a positive effect on patient care.

- Golightly and colleagues analyzed 28,081 drug information requests received from health care professionals and consumers by a regional drug information center over a two-year period.[5] In 76% of cases regarding medication problems, a beneficial effect was either documented or apparent from the nature of the initial call response. Medication-related problems were noted in 5,702 of 16,657 (34.2%) questions from consumers. Among these problems, 2,717, nearly 50%, constituted serious or potentially serious medication problems. More than 27% of calls regarding serious or potentially serious medication problems came from the elderly while 15% came from children or young adults. During the two years of the study, 1,434 medication problems were prevented or resolved in the elderly. Of these problems, 242 were potentially capable of leading to hospitalization if not corrected.

- A questionnaire was used by Hayman and colleagues to assess physician use of the drug information center at the Medical University of South Carolina.[6] Of the 100 physicians responding, 54 reported using the information received for direct patient care. In reply to the question, "Do you feel the drug information service has a noticeably favorable effect on patient care?", 55% replied "yes", 19% replied "no", and 26% were undecided. The "clinical significance of the information provided with respect to a particular patient's drug therapy" was rated "pertinent and of clinical importance" by 76%, "pertinent, but of little clinical importance" by 24%, "irrelevant" by 0%, and "incorrect or inaccurate" by 0%.

The various studies of the impact of drug information services suggest that the services provide useful patient care information to a variety of health professionals and to consumers. Most of the information appears to directly influence patient outcomes, especially if the information is patient-specific.

References

1. Smith JM. Drug information services -- an update. *Int Pharm Rev* 1988;1:1-4.
2. Walton CA. Education and training of the drug information specialist. *Drug Intell* 1967;1:133-7.
3. Rosenberg JM, Martino FP, Kirschenbaum HL, Robbins J. Pharmacist-operated drug information centers in the United States -- 1986. *Am J Hosp Pharm* 1987;44:337-44.
4. Cardoni AA, Thompson TJ. Impact of drug information services on patient care. *Am J Hosp Pharm* 1978;35:1233-7.
5. Golightly LK, Davis AG, Budwitz WJ, et al. Documenting the activity and effectiveness of a regional drug information center. *Am J Hosp Pharm* 1988;45:356-61.
6. Hayman JN, Brown TR, Smith MC, Liao W. Physician use and evaluation of a hospital-based drug information center. *Am J Hosp Pharm* 1978;35:1238-40.

Facilities

1. Location Within the Hospital

    a. Centralized

In order to conserve resources, drug information centers are usually centralized in an office. Unfortunately, this location is often geographically remote from the patient care area, making more productive, face-to-face dialogue inconvenient and telephone contact more common. To facilitate the response process to drug information questions, the drug information center should contain reference texts, journals, files, computers, telephones, and work space for staff and visitors.

    b. Decentralized

Mini-drug information centers may be set up in satellite pharmacies. Computerized databases may be accessible via computer terminals in any location, including patient care units and physicians' offices.

2. Regionalization/Communication

Because of the cost involved in establishing drug information centers (discussed later in this chapter) and the duplication of effort that may occur with drug information center staff in different institutions (e.g., in preparing Pharmacy and Therapeutics Committee reviews), it has been proposed that regional drug information centers should be established to perform functions in common to several institutions, or to answer drug information questions in geographic locations not otherwise served by a drug information center. A federally funded program established in the 1960s to explore this option in the United States was discontinued.[1] This concept was not readily accepted in the United States, particularly by the larger teaching hospitals, which tend to have unique patient populations and investigational drug treatment programs. However, economic pressures of the 1990's have caused some health care organizations to revisit this approach. Groups of hospitals and health maintenance organizations have banded together to enhance purchasing, research, and other activities, including drug information services. A central drug information office serves as a resource to the member institutions. An example is the University Hospital Consortium, a hospital group purchasing organization.

Regional drug information centers were established in the United Kingdom in the 1970s,[2] and still exist. Such centers have also been established in Canada.[3]

To enhance communication among individuals with common interests, electronic bulletin boards (EBB) have been developed.[4] These systems can be used for rapid communication to any number of other subscribers. For the cost of a computer, modem, communications software program, and applicable telephone charges, the user may connect with any of thousands of EBB in existence. Some EBB provide "conferences" for subscribers with specific shared interests. For example, PharmNet, developed by the American Society of Hospital Pharmacists (ASHP; 1-800-848-8980), has a Drug Information Conference. EBB with a focus on pharmacy or drug information are listed in Table 4-1.

Table 4-1.   Selected Electronic Bulletin Boards
_____

United States

- Black Bag BBS, Newark, DE
- CHOPIN, California Hospital Pharmacists Information Network, California Society of Hospital Pharmacists
- ClinNet, American College of Clinical Pharmacy, Kansas City, MO
- Darwin BBS, Darwin Systems, Inc., Rockville, MD
- Electronic Bulletin Board Service, Food and Drug Administration, Rockville , MD
- PediNet, Kapoor Center for Pediatric Drug Information (KCPDI) of the Pediatric Pharmacy Administrative Group (PPAG), Denver, CO
- PHARMLINE, American Association of Colleges of Pharmacy
- PharmNet, American Society of Hospital Pharmacists, Bethesda, MD
- ProComm, Datastorm Technology, Inc., Columbia, MO
- RBBS, Thomas D. Mack, Great Falls, VA
- Saint Peter Hospital BBS, Olympia, WA
- The F.I.X., The Formulary Information Exchange, The Formulary, Inc., Laguna, CA

Foreign

- Gezondheidszorg, Holland
- Health Professional BBS, Canada
- Intermedic, Canada
- IKM Opus, Germany
- Pharmacy OPUS, Australia
- SMA BBS, Singapore

_____

A unique forum for dissemination of drug information to consumers is through a computerized bulletin board service (BBS) on a local public access BBS. A group of pharmacists from the University Hospitals of Cleveland and PIRL Consultants of Cleveland have established "The Pharmacy", a BBS on the Cleveland FreeNet.[5] The service is also available to other health care providers and, in addition to providing a community service, enhances the visibility of pharmacists.

Personnel

1. Staffing

In order for users to believe that they can rely on the drug information center for service when needed, the center should have sufficient staffing to be immediately accessible during hours of operation. The center should also be available within a reasonable time period during evenings, weekends, or other hours when the center is not in operation. According to one survey, 99 of 130 (76%) drug information centers surveyed operated from 0900 to 1700 Monday through Friday.[6] Approximately 20% of the drug information centers responding to two surveys reported being available 24 hours per day.[6-7] A mechanism for emergency after-hours services was present in 47 centers in one survey.[7] Approximately 20% of the responding drug information centers also handle poison information inquires.[6-7]

2. Staff

With regard to drug information center staff, 44%, 9%, and 5% of the centers responding to one survey reported having one, two, or four full-time-equivalent pharmacist positions, respectively.[6] Pharmacy students, residents and fellows often receive training in a drug information center and must be adequately supervised. Secretarial support is essential, so that the professional drug information staff can focus on drug information activities rather than spending time on clerical functions.

3. Staff Profile

According to the results of a survey of drug information pharmacists at health care facilities, universities, and pharmaceutical companies published in 1992, most drug information pharmacists have been practicing for four years or less and are between the ages of 30 and 39.[8] More than half of the respondents have the Pharm.D. degree, and approximately 50% completed a postgraduate residency or fellowship. The respondents with advanced training reported more favorable professional outcomes in terms of career position, income, and job satisfaction. A career in drug information practice was selected because it included an opportunity for continued learning, job satisfaction, and regular work hours.

Funding

Major sources of funding for drug information centers in the United States are reported to be hospitals or medical centers (88% of drug information centers) and colleges or universities (32% of drug information centers).[9] Some drug information centers have made their services available for a fee to users including smaller nearby hospitals, law firms, medical advertising agencies, and others.[9-12] Charges are usually based on either the size of the subscribing institution (number of beds), the volume of information requests, or other services provided (e.g., newsletters, formulary reviews). The type of clients that may be charged a fee are listed in Table 4-2.[10]

Table 4-2.   Clients to Whom Drug Information Centers Provide Consultations for Fees[a]

Clients	Number (%) of Drug Information Centers Providing Consultations (n=23)
Attorneys or legal firms	17 (74)
Pharmaceutical firms or generic houses	7 (30)
Pharmaceutical advertising agencies	5 (22)
Symposia agencies	1 (4)
Others[b]	11 (48)

[a]   Adapted with permission from Crabbe SJ, Wordell CJ, Hopkins LE.   Fee-for-service activities provided by drug information centers. *Am J Hosp Pharm* 1988;45:1115-7.

[b]   Including hospital pharmacies (4), community pharmacies (2), insurance companies (1), a health clinic (1), hospital pharmacy network (1), state pharmaceutical association (1), and an on-line database vendor (1).

As indicated in Table 4-2, the primary source for paying professional fees are attorneys or legal firms. Although some drug information centers provide formal consultation programs to the legal profession,[13] the increased revenue generated must be weighed against the disadvantages of the time commitment and potential conflicts of interest.

Another source of funding based on fees is corporations, particularly pharmaceutical manufacturers. An example of this type of financial arrangement was described by Kimelblatt and colleagues.[14] Drug information services were marketed by this nonprofit group to profit-making firms such as symposia agencies, pharmaceutical advertising agencies, and television stations at a fee or "donation" of $75 per hour with a one-hour minimum.

In addition to institutional support or consultation fees, other sources of revenue are regional health authorities or professional groups such as pharmacists. For example, the Regional Center for Drug Information at the Milan (Italy) Mario Negri Institute for Pharmacological Research is funded by the Regional Health Authority and the National Research Council[15] and the drug information center at the Faculty of Pharmacy, University of Toronto, is funded by the Ontario College of Pharmacists and serves as a resource for pharmacists in Ontario.[16]

Over 70% of the drug information centers surveyed indicated that they charged a fee for written consultations (Table 4-3). Telephone consultations were the most common service for which a fee was charged. The next most common activity was literature searching.

Table 4-3.   Services Provided and Fees Charged by Drug Information Centers[a]

Service	Number (%) of Drug Information Centers Providing Services (n=23)	Number of Requests per Month	Time Required per Request (hours)	Hourly Fee ($)
Written consultation	16 (70)	1-5	1-8	25-150
Telephone consultation	15 (65)	1-150	0.8-8	0-100
Literature searching	12 (52)	<1-35	0.2-4	25-100[b]
Depositions	10 (43)	<1-1	1-15	40-150
Court appearances	9 (39)	<1	1-8	100-200
Document delivery	1 (4)	30	0.12	c

[a]   Adapted with permission from Crabbe SJ, Wordell CJ, Hopkins LE.   Fee-for-service activities provided by drug information centers. *Am J Hosp Pharm* 1988;45:1115-7.

[b]   A charge for on-line time may or may not be added to this fee.

[c]   The fee was $2 per document plus postage and photocopying expenses.

Expenses

Estimated drug information center operating expenses, as reported by drug information centers responding to the survey by Dombrowski and Visconti, are summarized in Table 4-4.[7] The sum of the mean annual expenses is $18,505. Several limitations to this figure should be noted: 1) many drug information centers had difficulty quantifying expenses exclusively associated with operation of the drug information center, 2) this total does not include salary or benefits, 3) the range of expenses in each category varied widely among drug information centers, and 4) the figures were collected in 1983 and should be adjusted for inflation.

Table 4-4.   Annual Expenses of Drug Information Centers[a]

Item	Number of Responses	Annual Expense ($)	
		Mean	Range
Subscriptions to journals, periodicals, and drug information systems	60	5,077	219-25,000
Fees for on-line computer services	32	1,007	50-10,000
New books	55	1,238	100- 6,864
New equipment	25	1,545	125-10,840
Photocopying and printing costs	38	2,793	100-15,000
Telephone	28	4,187	10-30,000
Postage	27	610	20- 6,000
Journal-binding costs	28	242	13- 750
Other	10	1,806	100- 6,700

[a]   Adapted with permission from Dombrowski SR, Visconti JA. National audit of drug information centers. *Am J Hosp Pharm* 1985;42:819-26.

References

1. Evens RP. The state of the art, and future directions, of drug information centers. *Pharm Int* 1985;19:74-7.
2. Leach FN. The regional drug information service: a factor in health care? *Br J Med* 1978;1:766-8.
3. Anon. Canadian drug information centres. *Can J Hosp Pharm* 1988;41:284-5.
4. Walkley S. Experience with electronic bulletin boards. *Am J Hosp Pharm* 1989;46:316-8.
5. Bednarczyk EM, Kyllonen K, Marcus P, Mendel S. Establishment of a drug information service on a public access computer bulletin board (abstract). *Pharmacotherapy* 1992;12:497.
6. Beaird SL, Coley RMR, Crea KA. Current status of drug information centers. *Am J Hosp Pharm* 1992;49:103-6.
7. Dombrowski SR, Visconti JA. National audit of drug information centers. *Am J Hosp Pharm* 1985;42:819-26.
8. Gong SD, Millares M, VanRiper KB. Drug information pharmacists at health-care facilities, universities, and pharmaceutical companies. *Am J Hosp Pharm* 1992;49:1121-30.
9. Rosenberg JM, Martino FP, Kirschenbaum HL, Robbins J. Pharmacist-operated drug information centers in the United States - 1986. *Am J Hosp Pharm* 1987;44:337-44.

10. Crabbe SJ, Wordell CJ, Hopkins LE. Fee-for-service activities provided by drug information centers. *Am J Hosp Pharm* 1988;45:1115-7.
11. Schweigert BF. Drug information services on a subscription basis. *Am J Hosp Pharm* 1976;33:823-7.
12. Skoutakis VA, Wojciechowski NJ, Carter CA, Hayes JM, Hudson BL, Martin JA. Drug information center network: need, effectiveness, and cost justification. *Drug Intell Clin Pharm* 1987;21:49-56.
13. Conner CS, Sawyer DR, Sbarbaro JA, Smolinske SC. Consultations with attorneys as a funding source for drug information centers. *Am J Hosp Pharm* 1982;39:1311-3.
14. Kimelblatt BJ, Kucich JM, Silverman HM, Simon GI. Marketing drug information to corporations. *Am J Hosp Pharm* 1982;39:313-4.
15. Kasilo O, Romero M, Bonati M, Tognoni G. Information on drug use in pregnancy from the viewpoint regional drug information centre. *Eur J Clin Pharmcol* 1988;35:447-53.
16. Murdoch LL. Foreign drug identification. *Drug Intell Clin Pharm* 1989;23:501-6.

Chapter 5   Poison Control Centers: Difference from Drug Information Centers

Poison control centers and drug information centers have overlapping responsibilities and resource needs, but are very different operations. A full discussion of poison control centers is beyond the scope of this book. In addition to the obvious predominance of toxicology, poisoning, or overdose questions received by a poison control center, the basic ways in which poison control centers differ from drug information centers are listed below:

1. Poison control centers receive a much higher number of calls from consumers.

2. Responses are usually needed more rapidly for poison control centers.

3. Some poison control centers (particularly those designated as Regional Poison Control Centers by the American Association of Poison Control Centers) are staffed 24 hours per day.

4. Poison control centers are often staffed by non-pharmacist poison information specialists.

Troutman and Wanke discussed the advantages and disadvantages of combining poison control centers and drug information centers.[1] The main advantages of combining these centers are 1) a reduction in overall operating costs by sharing personnel, resources, and space, and 2) improved access for the poison control center staff to the literature retrieval and analysis skills of the drug information pharmacist. Disadvantages include the difficulty of achieving maximum skills in both disciplines and the disruption of drug information projects due to the more emergent nature of poison information calls. These authors conclude that the advantages of combining poison control centers and drug information centers outweigh the disadvantages.

Reference

1. Troutman WG, Wanke LA. Advantages and disadvantages of combining poison control and drug information centers. *Am J Hosp Pharm* 1983;40:1219-22.

Assessments of quality assurance in drug information are difficult and evolving. Obstacles to these programs include manpower shortages, time requirements, and the lack of definitive methodology in this area.[1] Thompson and Heflin[2] list and discuss seven different methods for evaluating quality assurance in drug information centers and poison control centers:

1. Survey of user satisfaction
2. Assessment of the impact on patient care
3. Analysis of calls
4. Evaluation of completed drug information request forms
5. Committee review of the services
6. Internal review of the services
7. Telephone evaluation.

Uniformly accepted standards for quality assurance in drug information centers do not exist. A draft prepared by the American Society of Hospital Pharmacists (ASHP) Special Practice Group (SPG) on Drug Information has not yet been officially endorsed and issued by ASHP.[3] Some guidelines are listed in the accreditation standards for an ASHP-approved specialized residency in drug information (Appendix E).[4] Park and Benderev expanded on these guidelines to create criteria for their drug information center. The article is useful in not only providing the criteria that were derived, but in also describing the process used to create the quality assurance program for the drug information center.[5] Burkle suggested criteria, standards, and methods of assessment for a drug information service and related pharmacy functions.[6]

The experience of various researchers in the assessment of quality assurance in providing drug information is summarized below:

- Two preceptors used a validated quality assurance program to measure the performance of 22 doctor of pharmacy students in developing responses during a six-week drug information rotation.[7] At the start of the rotation, students were provided with a list of objective quality assurance guidelines (Appendix F) to follow when responding to drug information requests. Judgmental and nonjudgmental responses were evaluated separately using two five-point rating scales which were based on objective criteria (Appendix G). A score of 5 was excellent and 1 was considered unacceptable. A total of 660 (30 for each student) randomly selected responses were evaluated. A score of 5 was assigned to 52.3% of the responses evaluated, 4 to 29.1%, 3 to 12.9%, 2 to 4.5%, and 1 to 1.2%. No significant difference was noted in scores for judgmental versus nonjudgmental responses. Written responses, which were evaluated for accuracy, completeness, objectivity, and usefulness using an external quality assurance program, were assigned mean scores above 4 by the requestors of the information. Statistical testing of inter-rater reliability indicated moderate agreement between raters. A quality assurance program such as this appears to be an appropriate method for evaluating student performance and possibly improving the quality of drug information responses.

- At a Canadian drug information center, Repchinsky and colleagues developed criteria and standards for the drug information service and then measured performance against the standards.[8] Based on responses to questionnaires sent to users of the drug information center, satisfaction with the service did not meet the standards the center had set for itself. Parameters with a 100% standard and the actual positive response from users were "received in time to be of use" (91.8%), "accurate" (96.8%), "objective" (92.4%), and "complete" (75.9%). Though less than the pre-set standard of 80%, 69% of responses either had been used to alter patient therapy or could be used in future patient care. The authors identified several measures which could be taken to improve the center's performance or to improve data collection. Examples include making patient-specific requests a priority, keeping resources updated, providing written responses, and revising the standards or the quality assurance evaluation questionnaire.

  A later study by Repchinsky and colleagues compared performance for a hospital-based drug information center and a regional drug information center which shared the same space and resources.[9] Compliance with standards was similar for both drug information centers and close to the pre-set standards for timeliness (100%), accuracy (100%), objectivity (100%), completeness (80%), and use in patient care (70%). A significantly higher percentage of requestors to the hospital drug information center used the information to alter a patient's therapy, compared to callers to the regional drug information center (61.0% vs 37.6%, respectively), while significantly more of the callers to the regional drug information center indicated the information would be used to alter therapy in the future (35.3% vs 8.5%, respectively) (p <0.001).

- In 1977, Halbert and colleagues contacted 90 drug information centers by telephone with a standard question.[10] Most of the drug information centers provided acceptable responses, but a few provided erroneous or incomplete information. The authors point out the need for a system to "assure a minimum level of quality and competence". Such a system might include better trained staff, in-house review of drug information services, or following a more systematic and comprehensive approach when handling a drug information request.

- Gallo and colleagues had a panel of clinical pharmacists rate responses from 10 drug information centers for a single question.[11] The maximum possible rating was 100 (100%), based on directness of answer, applicability of answer, accuracy, and completeness. The range of rating was 23% to 84% (mean 62.2%). The "control" response, compiled by the investigators received a rating of 84%.

- Two methods of quality assurance assessment were used by Johnson and Dupuis: a user survey and committee review.[1] Surveys were sent to a total of 69 drug information requestors for whom the drug information response involved literature assessment during the study year. This group was not representative of the drug information user population; a higher percentage of user surveys was sent to physicians (79%), while only 38% of the total (oral and written) drug information requests were from physicians. Using a 10-point scale, the users rated the responses very high on all measures: timing (mean 9.2 +/- 1.1 on a scale of 10); usefulness (9.3 +/- 1.0); completeness (9.5 +/- 0.7); therapy change (8.3 +/- 3.0); effect on patient care (8.8 +/- 1.7); overall rating (9.3 +/- 1.2). The ratings may have been artificially high because the visual analog scale designed for user ratings is not clearly presented and appears to force selections at either end of the scale. An additional problem with the reliability of the users' responses was that the question could have been answered as much as one year before the survey was sent.

The committee review process resulted in even higher ratings (mean 0.934 to 0.994, with the highest possible score being 1.0) for a different combination of factors: literature correlation/condensation, data documentation, literature evaluation, conclusion, references, organization, terminology, and sentence structure. The review committee consisted of two physicians (one of whom stopped participating due to time constraints) and two pharmacists who were not affiliated with the drug information service. The authors commented that the committee review method is extremely time consuming, and they plan to use it in the future only if quality problems are found by future user surveys.

- Methods similar to those of Johnson and Dupuis (peer evaluation and user survey) were used by other investigators, who studied the quality of drug information responses provided by staff pharmacists working outside of a drug information center.[12] The peer reviewers found documentation criteria to be met for more than 90% of requests, except for documentation of the requestor's name (73%), location / telephone / pager (65%), and references sent (79%). Assessment criteria were met at the following incidences: adequate patient information obtained, 82%; appropriate clinical considerations applied, 88%; response met standard, 85%; appropriate references used, 90%. As assessed by the auditors (not the users) with a five-point scale, the mean potential of the response to influence patient outcome was 3.7, and the mean potential to influence drug selection or administration in patient care areas was 3.3. Sixty-seven percent of responses were considered to require judgment.

The users rated drug information services provided by the staff pharmacists as outstanding (22%), above average (35%), and average (30%). In comparison, ratings of the drug information center in the same hospital were outstanding (24%), above average (55%), average (14%), and below average (2%), using a similar questionnaire.

References

1. Johnson N, Dupuis LL. A quality assurance audit of a drug information service. *Can J Hosp Pharm* 1989;42:57-61.
2. Thompson DF, Heflin NR. Quality assurance in drug information and poison centers: a review. *Hosp Pharm* 1985;20:758-60.
3. American Society of Hospital Pharmacists SPG on Drug and Poison Information Practice. Draft of minimum standards for drug information centers and guidelines for quality assurance for drug information services. Bethesda, MD: American Society of Hospital Pharmacists, 1993.
4. American Society of Hospital Pharmacists. ASHP supplemental standard and learning objectives for residency training in drug information practice. *Am J Hosp Pharm* 1982;39:1970-2.

5. Park BA, Benderev KP. Quality assurance program for a drug information center. *Am J Hosp Pharm* 1985;42:2180-4.
6. Burkle WS. Developing a quality assurance program for clinical services. *Hosp Pharm* 1982;17:125-47.
7. Restino MSR, Knodel LC. Drug information quality assurance program used to appraise students' performance. *Am J Hosp Pharm* 1992;49:1425-9.
8. Repchinsky CA, Masuhara EJ. Quality assurance program for a drug information center. *Drug Intell Clin Pharm* 1987;21:816-20.
9. Repchinsky C, Godbout L, Tierney M. A quality assurance audit for a regional and a hospital drug information service. *Can J Hosp Pharm* 1988;41:267-9.
10. Halbert MR, Kelly WN, Miller DE. Drug information centers: lack of generic equivalence. *Drug Intell Clin Pharm* 1977;11:728-35.
11. Gallo GR, VanderZanden JA, Wertheimer AI. Anonymous peer review of answers received from drug information centres. *J Clin Hosp Pharm* 1985;10:397-401.
12. Sketris IS, Bishop A, Somers E, Baker GR. Developing a quality assurance program for drug information requests answered by staff pharmacists. *Drug Inf J* 1989;23:327-34.

Ethics

Some drug information questions raise ethical issues which should be considered prior to providing a response. Arnold and colleagues found that the most frequently asked drug information questions raising ethical issues were drug identification questions, particularly when asked by consumers wanting to identify another person's medications.[1] For example, parents often find drugs in their children's clothing and want to have the product identified. Ethical issues raised in this situation include confidentiality, invasion of privacy, and drug abuse.

Other types of questions which involved ethical issues include asking pharmacists to assess a physician's recommendation, public health or legal issues, therapeutic issues in which the professional and private ethics of the pharmacist may be in conflict, and questions from belligerent or psychologically impaired callers (e.g., suicidal person asking how much is a lethal dose).[1-2]

The frequency of calls involving ethical issues was greater for calls from consumers (29 of 744 total calls) than for calls from health care professionals (14 calls from pharmacists, 2 from nurses, and 1 from a physician).[1]

Drug information providers should give some consideration to the moral, legal, and consistency aspects of responding to questions that raise ethical issues. For further information regarding ethics, a list of 31 selected literature citations on ethics may be consulted.[2]

Liability

Clear answers are not available on the potential liability of drug information providers. Clark and colleagues[3] offer the following suggestions to avoid or reduce liability risk:

1. Obtain peer concurrence
2. Avoid violation of statutes and regulations
3. Comply with professional standards and guidelines
4. Follow set policies and procedures
5. Document services
6. Seek professional support
7. Obtain adequate professional liability insurance.

References

1. Arnold RM, Nissen JC, Campbell NA. Ethical issues in a drug information center. *Drug Intell Clin Pharm* 1987;21:1008-11.

2. Uretsky SD, Kelly WN, Veatch RM. Pharmacist's responsibility for providing drug information to be used for questionable purposes. *Am J Hosp Pharm* 1992;49:1725-30.

3. Clark TT, White BD, Hamner ME. Liability of drug information centers. *US Pharm* 1982;7:39-42,56.

References

1.   Reference Texts

The references most commonly available in drug information centers in the United States are listed in Table 8-1[1-2] and those most frequently consulted in European drug information centers are listed in Table 8-2.[3]

Table 8-1.   Reference Texts Commonly Available in United States Drug Information Centers[a]

Reference Text	(%)[b] Drug Information Centers (n=127)
Facts and Comparisons[c]	100
Martindale: The Extra Pharmacopoeia[c]	100
AHFS Drug Information[c]	99
Handbook of Injectable Drugs[c]	99
Physicians' Desk Reference[c]	99
The Pharmaceutical Basis of Therapeutics[c]	99
Clinical Toxicology of Commercial Products	98
Drug Interactions (Hansten)	98
Handbook of Nonprescription Drugs[c]	98
Merck Index	96
Harrison's Principles of Internal Medicine	95
Remington's Pharmaceutical Sciences[c]	95
American Drug Index	94
Applied Therapeutics[c]	94
Handbook of Antimicrobial Therapy	91
Handbook of Clinical Drug Data[c]	91
Meyler's Side Effects of Drugs	89
United States Pharmacopeia/National Formulary	88
AMA Drug Evaluations	87
Handbook of Poisoning (Driesbach)	87
USP DI	87

[a]   Adapted with permission from Rosenberg JM, Martino FP, Kirschenbaum HL, Robbins J. Pharmacist-operated drug information centers in the United States -- 1986. *Am J Hosp Pharm* 1987;44:337-44.

[b]   Rounded to the nearest whole number

[c]   Available in 117 or more of the 130 (90%) centers that responded to a 1990 survey[1]

Table 8-2.   Reference Texts Frequently Consulted in European Drug Information Centers[a]

Name of Reference Text[b]	Number of Drug Information Centers[c]
Martindale: The Extra Pharmacopoeia	18
The Pharmaceutical Basis of Therapeutics	
(Goodman and Gilman)	11
Meyler's Side Effects of Drugs	10
AHFS Drug Information 86	
(American Society of Hospital Pharmacists)	8
Drug Treatment	
(GS Avery)	6
Formularies	3
A Manual of Adverse Drug Reactions	
(JP Griffith and PF D'Arcy)	3
Iatrogenic Diseases	
(PF D'Arcy and JP Griffith)	3
Index Nominum	
(Swiss Pharmaceutical Society)	2
Drug Interactions	
(IH Stockley)	2

[a]   Adapted with permission from Maguire ME, D'Arcy PF. Present drug information services in Europe including 'The two pharmacists of Verona'. *Int Pharm J* 1990;4:49-56.
[b]   Authors/editors or publisher appear in parentheses
[c]   There were 29 drug information centers that responded to this survey.

2.   Journals, Periodicals, and Drug Information Systems

Table 8-3 lists the percentage of drug information centers in the United States subscribing to various journals, periodicals, and drug information systems.[2] Table 8-4 lists the journals most frequently consulted by European drug information centers or associated libraries.[3]

Table 8-3. Journals, Newsletters, and Drug Information Systems Commonly Available in Drug Information Centers in the United States[a]

Name of Reference	(%)[b] Drug Information Centers (n=127)
Journals	
American Journal of Hospital Pharmacy	100
Drug Intelligence and Clinical Pharmacy (*DICP Annals of Pharmacotherapy*)	98
Clinical Pharmacy	96
Hospital Formulary	96
Drug Therapy	92
New England Journal of Medicine	91
Journal of the American Medical Association	84
Newsletters	
The Medical Letter	98
FDA Drug Bulletin	87
Clin-Alert	67
Facts and Comparisons Newsletter	67
Drug Information Systems	
Iowa Drug Information Service	80
Index Medicus	58
Drugdex	54
Identidex	54
Poisindex	53
International Pharmaceutical Abstracts	43
Unlisted Drugs	35
Paul de Haen Information Systems	31

[a] Adapted with permission from Rosenberg JM, Martino FP, Kirschenbaum HL, Robbins J. Pharmacist-operated drug information centers in the United States -- 1986. *Am J Hosp Pharm* 1987;44:337-44.

[b] Rounded to nearest whole number

Table 8-4.   Journals Frequently Consulted in European Drug Information Centers or Associated Libraries[a]

Name of Journal	Number of Drug Information Centers[b]
Lancet	13
New England Journal of Medicine	10
Drugs	9
British Medical Journal	7
Drug Intelligence and Clinical Pharmacy	7
Journal of the American Medical Association	5
Inpharma	5
American Journal of Hospital Pharmacy	4
Drug and Therapeutics Bulletin	3
Clinical Pharmacy	2

[a]   Adapted with permission from Maguire ME, D'Arcy PF. Present drug information services in Europe including 'The two pharmacists of Verona'. *Int Pharm J* 1990;4:49-56.

[b]   There were 29 drug information centers that responded to this survey.

3.   Use of Computers and Selected Drug Information Systems

The emergence of computer software for enhancing clinical decision making has gained applicability and acceptance among drug information practitioners. In the United States, 96% of drug information centers use computers in some aspect of their services.[1] In one survey completed in 1986, computers were reportedly used for on-line searching (76%), record keeping (60%), storage and retrieval of data (48%), pharmacokinetic calculations (40%), and word processing (30%).[2] Computerized drug information centers which used commercial databases preferred MEDLINE (76%), followed by *International Pharmaceutical Abstracts* (38%), TOXLINE (16%), and *Excerpta Medica* (11%).[2] In a survey conducted by Dombrowski and Visconti in 1985, the monthly average number of computer-assisted literature searches by drug information centers in the United States was 8.8 +/- 17.5 (range 0-150).[4] Data collected five years later in 1990 indicate that 74% (96 of 130) of drug information centers perform computer-assisted literature searches with a median of 5 to 10 searches performed monthly.[1]

Based on a crossover comparison of the drug information on-line database vendors Dialog Information Services (includes *Excerpta Medica* and EMBASE) and the National Library of Medicine's MEDLARS (Medical Literature Analysis and Retrieval System; includes MEDLINE, TOXLINE, TOXLIT), Rovers and colleagues[5] have developed the following guidelines for searching databases to respond to routine drug information requests:

- Search nonroyalty MEDLARS databases first as they are clinically comparable at a significantly lower cost. The high cost of EMBASE may limit its value for routine drug information use.
- For toxicology or adverse drug reaction information search MEDLINE first, then investigate TOXLINE, and lastly TOXLIT.
- Use EMBASE after MEDLARS because it has the capability to provide responses to routine requests that remain unresolved following exhaustion of all MEDLARS databases.
- Consider the following cost containment strategies:
  -plan the search before connecting to the database
  -search during "off hours" (5 pm to 10 am Monday through Friday)
  -print offline
  -use LOGOFF HOLD (Dialog Information Services)
  -use savesearch (MEDLARS)
  -use a contract prepaid subscription plan (Dialog Information Services).

An emerging alternative to on-line database searching is the use of compact discs (CDs) such as MEDLINE on CD-ROM. The advantages of CDs include greater flexibility in use and lack of on-line charges, which may result in more comprehensive literature searches. Searching the literature using CDs is more desirable for inexperienced users because of the lower time and cost constraints. The major disadvantage is the higher initial costs of the CDs and the hardware needed to use them.[5-6] Another CD drug information resource is the Drug Information Source™.[7] Produced by the Cambridge Information Group and available through the Database Services Division of the American Society of Hospital Pharmacists, this resource combines the *AHFS Drug Information®*, *Handbook on Injectable Drugs*, and *International Pharmaceutical Abstracts®* (*IPA*) on one CD that is updated quarterly. *IPA* is also available alone on CD. *AHFS Drug Information®* is available along with texts including *Scientific American Medicine* and other publications on STAT!-Ref, a CD produced by Teton Data Systems and available through ASHP.

Category-specific drug information systems have also emerged as a convenient tool in drug information centers. Available through the National Library of Medicine are three AIDS databases (AIDSLINE, AIDSDRUGS, AIDSTRIALS) and an oncology database (CANCERLIT).[8] An IBM-compatible drug information system that provides information on the use of drugs during pregnancy and lactation is available by subscription through the Drug Information Center at Monash Medical Center, Clayton, Victoria, Australia.[9] A number of computerized drug interaction screening programs exist including Medicom Micro Plus, Medical Letter, S-O-A-P, Drug Interactions (Hansten), Drug Therapy Screening Systems (DTSS), and RxTriage, each with specific advantages and disadvantages.[10]

Among European drug information centers, a 1989 study indicated that 95% reported having access to computers either in the drug information center or in an associated library.[3] The number of European drug information centers subscribing to various information systems is provided in Table 8-5.[3] Table 8-6 lists vendors and databases available to many European drug information centers.[3]

Table 8-5.   Drug Information Systems Available in European Drug Information Centers (1989)[a]

Name of Information System	Number of Drug Information Centers[b]
Iowa Drug Information Service (IDIS)	17
Pharmaceutical Societies Library Service (e.g., Royal Pharmaceutical Society of Great Britain)	15
Associated libraries	12
Inpharma	11
Formularies (e.g., British National Formulary)	9
Drugdex	6
Pharmline fiche (Great Britain National Health Service)	6
Excerpta Medica (e.g., Clinical Pharmacology)	4
Current Contents (e.g., Clinical Medicine)	4
International Pharmaceutical Abstracts	4
Pharmacy School Information Services	4
Medical specialists	3
Scrip	3
Paul de Haen (Drugs in Research)	2

[a]   Adapted with permission from Maguire ME, D'Arcy PF. Present drug information services in Europe including 'The two pharmacists of Verona'. *Int Pharm J* 1990;4:49-56.

[b]   There were 29 drug information centers that responded to this survey.

Table 8-6.   On-line Computer Facilities Available for Access by Drug Information Pharmacists in Europe[a]

Vendors

Data-Cantralen	(Danish)
Data Star	(Swiss)
Dialogue	(USA)
DIMDI	(German)
IRS-Dialtech	(European Space Agency) British
Pergamon-Orbit	(Maxwell Communications International)
STN	(German)
Telesystem-Questral	(French)

Databases

DRUGLINE
EMBASE
Martindale
MEDLINE
PHARMLINE
RISKLINE
TOXLINE

Others

MEDLINE on Compact Discs (e.g., use EBSCO C-D ROM discs)
Prestel

[a]   Adapted with permission from Maguire ME, D'Arcy PF. Present drug information services in Europe including 'The two pharmacists of Verona'. *Int Pharm J* 1990;4:49-56.

4.   Storage and Retrieval of Drug Information Responses

In a 1985 survey, most drug information centers (75%) reported that they maintain a system for documentation and retrieval of responses to previously answered drug information questions, either by keeping a chronological log or by filing in some other manner.[4] Computers may be used for this purpose, as described by Fischer.[11]

Resource Materials

A complete listing and description of useful drug information resource materials is beyond the scope of this book. An excellent book by Snow, a pharmaceutical librarian, is recommended for those seeking this kind of aid.[12] A classic drug information *Guide* by Sewell has proven to be invaluable by students and practitioners for many years.[13] For those interested in medical librarianship, a classic *Reader* presents the philosophy of medical librarianship.[14]

Descriptions of drug information references, while useful as a starting point, are inadequate for making decisions about what references to purchase for one's own library. Copies of the references should be examined first-hand, whenever possible.

References

1. Beaird SL, Coley RMR, Crea KA. Current status of drug information centers. *Am J Hosp Pharm* 1992;49:103-6.
2. Rosenberg JM, Martino FP, Kirschenbaum HL, Robbins J. Pharmacist-operated drug information centers in the United States -- 1986. *Am J Hosp Pharm* 1987;44:337-44.
3. Maguire ME, D'Arcy PF. Present drug information services in Europe including 'The two pharmacists of Verona'. *Int Pharm J* 1990;4:49-56.
4. Dombrowski SR, Visconti JA. National audit of drug information centers. *Am J Hosp Pharm* 1985;42:819-26.
5. Rovers JP, Janosik JE, Souney PF. Crossover comparison of drug information online database vendors: Dailog and MEDLARS. *Ann Pharmacother* 1993;27:634-9.
6. Searching MEDLINE. *Lancet* 1988;2:663-4.
7. Tousignaut DR, Moss SK. *International Pharmaceutical Abstracts* on CD ROM. *Am J Hosp Pharm* 1990;47:1519, 22.
8. Minor JR. What online computer resources are available for obtaining AIDS-related information? *Am J Hosp Pharm* 1990;47:1130.
9. James A. Information on drug use during pregnancy and lactation. *Am J Hosp Pharm* 1990;47:1017.
10. Jankel CA, Martin BC. Evaluation of six computerized drug interaction screening programs. *Am J Hosp Pharm* 1992;49:1430-5.
11. Fischer JM. Dibase: a unique on-line real-time system for storage and retrieval of data from drug information requests. *Drug Inf J* 1980;14:107-12.
12. Snow B. Drug information: a guide to current resources. Medical Library Association, Inc., Chicago, Illinois, 1989.
13. Sewell W. Guide to drug information. Drug Intelligence Publications, Inc., Hamilton, IL, 1976.
14. Sewell W. Reader in medical librarianship. Reader series in library and information Science. NCR/Microcard Editions, Washington, D.C., 1973.

SECTION II   *Responding to Drug Information Questions*

As described in Chapter 2, drug information centers may serve several different functions. The one function which is most universally provided by drug information centers (and is implicit in the definition of drug information) is that of responding to individuals' specific drug information questions. Little new information on the systematic approach to answering drug information questions has been published since the publication of "Principles of Drug Information Services" by Watanabe and Conner in 1978. The process is best learned through experience, rather than reading. Guidance is provided in Chapters 9, 10, and 11.

Chapter 9   Question Analysis

---

1.   Assessing Drug Information Needs: What is being asked?

Assessment of the drug information question is an art as much as a science. Almost without exception, the question as it is originally worded is different than (or only a subset of) the question that really needs to be answered. With patience, intelligence, and sensitivity, the drug information provider can obtain additional information from the requestor which will enable a much more meaningful exchange of information, resulting in greater patient benefit.

Before determining the questions needed to obtain the appropriate background information (explained later in this chapter), it is helpful to classify the original request into some general categories.

2.   How is a Request Classified?

a.   By requestor

With some notable exceptions, the level of detail required by some requestors can be anticipated. Physicians tend to be interested in more technical responses than nurses. However, the background of the specific individual must always be taken into consideration. For example, a nurse working in a hemodialysis unit may have a far more sophisticated understanding of the renal excretion of drugs than might a neurosurgeon whose practice does not usually involve this topic.

b.   By category of information

There are two primary reasons why it is often helpful to categorize information requests according to the type of information requested (e.g., drug interaction, adverse drug reaction, parenteral compatibility). One reason is to aid the drug information provider in steering the search to those references which are particularly suited for a certain type of question.

Another reason to categorize the question by type of information is to aid in the selection of background questions that are helpful for eliciting additional information. For example, typical background questions to ask regarding the dosing of an antibiotic concern the age and weight of the patient, liver or kidney function, the site of the infection, and the suspected organism(s).

3.   Categories of Drug Information Questions and Corresponding Background Questions to Ask

With practice and experience, most drug information specialists develop a very rapid, efficient, and thorough system of gathering the relevant information required to categorize information requests and to elicit the additional background information required.

a. Therapeutic use

As indicated in Rosenberg's surveys (Table 2-1), questions on "therapeutic use" compose the largest single category of requests received by drug information centers.[1] Generally, questions in this category have one of two orientations:

1) drug-oriented (concerning the use of a particular drug)

What is Drug A used for? Is Drug A useful to treat Disease X?

2) disease or problem-oriented (concerning the treatment of a disease or problem)

What can/should be used to treat Disease X? What is the drug treatment of choice for Disease X?

If a specific patient is involved, the following information may be needed in order to provide the most useful response:

- patient age, weight, sex, race/ethnic origin
- medical problems
- organ function, particularly kidney and liver
- concomitant medications (prescription and over-the-counter), including dose, duration, route, indication for use
- history of medication allergies or adverse drug reactions.

The selection of therapy should be based on careful consideration of factors such as efficacy, safety, convenience (e.g., availability, frequency of administration), and cost (including associated costs resulting from the choice of therapy, such as extra lab tests needed for appropriate patient monitoring).

b. Drug dosage

Background information is extremely important to obtain for many drug dosage questions. For example, the answer to the question, "What is the recommended dose of indomethacin?" is dramatically different if the patient is a neonate with patent ductus arteriosus who is to receive the drug intravenously, versus an adult patient who is to receive the drug orally for severe rheumatoid arthritis.

Information to collect for drug dosage questions includes:

- patient size: some drugs are dosed on the basis of weight (usually expressed in kg) or body surface area (BSA, expressed in m^2)
- patient age: very young and very old patients metabolize some drugs differently than most adults
- patient gender
- function of significant organs, especially kidney and liver, because these organs are responsible for the majority of drug elimination

- the indication or condition being treated
- the desired route of administration, especially if the drug's bioavailability varies significantly by dosage form or route of delivery

c. Drug identification and availability

Considerable effort can be saved by taking the time to obtain the following information before searching through references to identify drugs:

- What is the drug's country of origin?
- How did the drug come to the attention of the requestor? Did the patient bring it in? Read about it in a journal?
- For what indication(s) is the drug used?
- Is the name a trade name, generic name, chemical name, or slang name? How sure is the requestor of the spelling?
- Is the drug available by prescription or over-the-counter?
- How does the drug appear? Are there any markings which may indicate the manufacturer or drug strength?
- How old is the drug thought to be? Might it no longer be marketed?
- Is the requestor interested in identifying an equivalent product which may be available?

Note that the official nonproprietary name for a drug may differ in different countries. In the United States, official nonproprietary drug names are assigned by the United States Adopted Names (USAN) Council. Other commonly encountered official names are the British Approved Name (BAN) and the International Nonproprietary Name (INN). The official name for a drug is important to consider when using drug information references from countries with different official naming systems, so that the appropriate term is used when using the references' indexes. The *European Drug Index*, published by the European Society of Clinical Pharmacy, provides a reference list of approximately 18,000 drugs marketed in 11 European countries. *Index Nominum International Drug Directory*, distributed worldwide, is an indispensable resource for identifying drug products available in 27 countries worldwide. Among other foreign information sources useful in identifying drugs are the following: *Martindale: The Extra Pharmacopoeia*, an English language text covering most of the drugs used clinically worldwide; *Diccionario de Especialidades Farmaceuticas*, a Spanish language compilation of drugs available in Mexico; *Dictionnaire Vidal*, a French language comprehensive listing of pharmaceuticals prescribed in France; *Rote Liste*, a German language listing of drugs approved by the Federal Association of Pharmaceutical Industry in Germany; and *Repertorio Farmaceutico Italiano*, an Italian language listing of approximately 1,200 drugs.

Prescriber requests for importing foreign drugs or biologics that appear to be best for a particular patient should be handled on the basis of the guidelines developed by the Food and Drug Administration (FDA) and the organization's institutional review board (IRB).[2] Requests for foreign drug or biologic importation require completion of the most recent versions of FDA forms 1571 or 1572, which are available by contacting the FDA Center for Drug Evaluation and Research (CDER).

d.   Adverse drug reactions (ADRs)

Questions concerning ADRs usually occur in one of two situations:

1)   a patient has experienced a problem and the requestor is attempting to establish a causal relationship between the problem and one of the patient's medications.

2)   a particular medication has not yet been given to a patient, but is being considered, and the requestor wishes to know more about the ADR profile or likelihood of the drug causing a problem in the specific patient, before deciding to prescribe, dispense, or administer the medication.

In the first situation, several background questions should be asked to assess the causal relationship between the potential ADR or medical event and the medication, as well as to determine how to best manage the problem:

- What signs and symptoms were associated with the event? How severe was it?
- When did the event occur relative to when the medication was administered? How long did it last? Have the signs and symptoms associated with the event resolved?
- What other medications was the patient taking? (Determine if drugs which may cause the same ADR or drug-drug interactions were also taken.)
- Does the patient have a prior history of allergy or reaction to the same or related medications? Does any family member?
- Does the patient have other medical problems that may contribute to the problem?
- How has the event been managed so far? What was the response to this intervention?

Algorithms have been published for establishing a possible, probable, or definite causal relationship for ADRs,[3-5] although their use is controversial.[6] A comparison of three algorithms found that of Naranjo[4] (Table 9-1), which is labeled as an ADR Probability Scale, to be preferable because it is simple, rapid to use, and it agrees well with a more sophisticated algorithm.[7]

Case and Oszko used an algorithm to evaluate 44 published ADR reports.[8] The authors objectively evaluated the reported assessments of the drug-adverse effect relationship and then compared them with assessments produced by an algorithm.[8] The assessments of both reviewers concurred with those of the authors in 17 (39%) of the cases. In 34 (77%) cases, at least one reviewer's assessment coincided with that of the authors. All three evaluators arrived at disparate conclusions in only two (5%) cases. The variability between assessments of a potential adverse effect may be considerable as a result of differing levels of clinical experience between reviewers, clinical judgment questions in the algorithms, and lack of adequate information in some of the published reports for the reader to assess causality. The methods used to assess an ADR should be included in ADR reports to assist clinicians in evaluating the case report.

ADRs should be reported to the FDA or to the manufacturer (who will forward the report to the FDA) using FDA form 3500 (Appendix D).[9] ADRs may also be reported to the United States Pharmacopeia (USP) Practitioners' Reporting Network (PRN) using the Drug Product Problem reporting form (Appendix D). The USP-PRN forwards the information received in each report to the FDA and the product manufacturer. An advantage of reporting the event to the manufacturer is that information may be obtained regarding previous similar reports, if any.

Table 9-1.   ADR Probability Scale[a]

To assess the adverse drug reaction, please answer the following questionnaire and give the pertinent score.

		Yes	No	Do Not Know
1.	Are there previous conclusive reports on this reaction?	+1	0	0
2.	Did the adverse event appear after the suspected drug was administered?	+2	-1	0
3.	Did the adverse reaction improve when the drug was discontinued or a *specific* antagonist was administered?	+1	0	0
4.	Did the adverse reaction reappear when the drug was readministered?	+2	-1	0
5.	Are there alternative causes (other than the drug) that could on their own have caused the reaction?	-1	+2	0
6.	Did the reaction reappear when a placebo was given?	-1	+1	0
7.	Was the drug detected in the blood (or other fluids) in concentrations known to be toxic?	+1	0	0
8.	Was the reaction more severe when the dose was increased, or less severe when the dose was decreased?	+1	0	0
9.	Did the patient have a similar reaction to the same or similar drugs in *any* previous exposure?	+1	0	0
10.	Was the adverse event confirmed by any objective evidence?	+1	0	0
	Total Score			

[a]   Adapted with permission from Naranjo CA, Busto A, Sellers EM, et al. A method for estimating the probability of adverse drug reactions. *Clin Pharmacol Ther* 1981;30:239-45.

e.   Pharmaceutical compatibility/stability

Factors to consider when assessing a pharmaceutical compatibility or stability problem include the following:

- route and site of administration
- timing of doses
- manufacturer or brand of product (data from one brand may not be extrapolated to other brands)

f.   Toxicology/poisoning

It is important to get a sense of the appropriate urgency with which the information is needed for toxicology and poisoning questions. Among the possible relevant questions in this type of inquiry are the following:

- Is a patient involved? (Or is the question one of academic interest, or does the call involve an animal such as a pet?)
- How much time has elapsed since the exposure?
- What is the drug, chemical, or plant involved?
- How much was ingested, inhaled, or received by another route? Clues: how much was dispensed in the original container? how much is remaining in the container? how much is still in the child's mouth? how much has spilled in the area?
- Confirm the route of exposure.
- What is the patient's age and weight?
- Were any other compounds also ingested, such as alcohol?
- What symptoms have been reported?
- What treatments have been attempted?
- Does the patient have any other medical problems? What is the current status of the patient's renal and hepatic function?

g.   Drug-drug, drug-food, or drug-laboratory test interactions

Among the possible relevant questions in this type of inquiry are the following:

- Has the suspected reaction already occurred? If so, what were the consequences? (useful for determining how to manage the patient)
- What specific drugs, foods, or laboratory tests (including test methods) were involved?
- What doses were used? For how long was the patient treated? What was the time course of events?

h.   Therapeutic drug monitoring/pharmacokinetics

Among the possible relevant questions in this type of inquiry are the following:

- What is the indication for which the drug is being used?
- What organism(s) are involved? (for anti-infective agents)

- What is the site of infection? (for anti-infective agents)
- What route of administration?
- What is the time course of drug administration and sampling of specimens?
- Is the recording accurate for dose and sampling times?

i.   Drug use in pregnancy/teratogenicity[11]

Among the possible relevant questions in this type of inquiry are the following:

- What agent was used? How much was used? When during the pregnancy was the agent used? What was the duration of exposure to the agent?
- What is the age, gravida, parity, and date of last menstrual period of the pregnant woman exposed to the agent?

References

1.   Rosenberg JM, Martino FP, Kirschenbaum HL, Robbins J. Pharmacist-operated drug information centers in the United States--1986. *Am J Hosp Pharm* 1987;44:337-44.
2.   Shirk M, Hale KN. Obtaining drugs from foreign markets. *Am J Hosp Pharm* 1992;49:2731-9.
3.   Kramer MS, Leventhal JM, Hutchinson TA, Feinstein AR. An algorithm for the operational assessment of adverse drug reactions. I. Background, description, and instructions for use. *JAMA* 1979;242:623-32.
4.   Naranjo CA, Busto A, Sellers EM, et al. A method for estimating the probability of adverse drug reactions. *Clin Pharmacol Ther* 1981;30:239-45.
5.   Jones JK. Adverse drug reactions in the community health setting: approaches to recognizing, counseling, and reporting. *Fam Comm Health* 1982;5:58-67.
6.   Hutchinson TA, Lane DA. Standardized methods of causality assessment for suspected adverse drug reactions (editorial). *J Chron Dis* 1986;39:857-60.
7.   Michel DJ, Knodel LC. Comparison of three algorithms used to evaluate adverse drug reactions. *Am J Hosp Pharm* 1986;43:1709-14.
8.   Case B, Oszko MA. Use of an algorithm to evaluate published reports of adverse drug reactions. *Am J Hosp Pharm* 1991;48:121-2.
9.   Kessler DA. Introducing MEDWatch. A new approach to reporting medication and device adverse effects and product problems. *JAMA* 1993;269:2765-8.
10. Department of Health and Human Services, Food and Drug Administration. Form for reporting serious adverse events and product problems with human drug and biological products and devices; availability. *Federal Register* 1993;58(105):31596-610.
11. LaFauce L, Williams CA, Ausbon W, Moffett M. The Florida teratogen information service. *Florida Med J* 1988;75:814-6.

The next step in answering a drug information question is to systematically search the available resources for relevant information.

1. *How to Develop and Conduct a Systematic Search*

   a. From general to specific

   With the abundance of information available, one could spend a large amount of time searching for information to respond to a drug information request. Practical considerations require that the searcher have some organized plan for the information search. This plan should include guidelines regarding when to search further and when to stop searching. In general, the recommended approach for locating appropriate information is to start with the most general references and move progressively toward the more detailed references, as required by the sophistication of the question or the needs of the requestor. In this manner, the responder can obtain a general overview of the information quickly and be able to put isolated details or conflicting findings into more appropriate perspective.

   b. Use specialized references

   Specialized references have been developed for locating information quickly on certain types of drug information questions. After determining the type of question that is being asked (see Chapter 9), it is often most efficient to go directly to these specialized references. For example, if a question concerns a drug interaction, the most efficient search process would probably involve consulting a drug interaction textbook, followed by a drug interaction newsletter, an indexing and abstracting service, and recent primary literature (see section on Classification of Information Sources). Depending on the length of time that the interaction has been studied and the degree of detail appropriate to the requestor, a suitable answer may be obtained from the first reference checked, the drug interaction text. However, if a general drug information compendium had been consulted first, information on drug interactions may have been missing, incomplete, or outdated, resulting in a waste of the time spent using that reference.

   c. Know your time frame

   Differences in the detail or comprehensiveness of responses are to be expected when short or long periods of time are available for researching the question and formulating a response. If the time frame given is too short to provide a completely researched answer and the responder is pressed to give a tentative response, it should be clearly communicated that the answer is tentative and that additional time will be needed for a complete response. The responder should estimate how much time will be required for the complete response and followup within that time period.

d. Adjust the search course as needed

If, in the process of researching a question, additional points emerge as potentially important, the search strategy should be adjusted to accommodate those new aspects.

2. *Classification of Information Sources*

The scientific literature is commonly classified as "primary", "secondary", or "tertiary." The term "primary literature" is used to describe published data such as original research articles or case reports. Primary literature provides the most detail on study design and results, compared with secondary or tertiary literature. "Secondary literature" refers to indexing and abstracting services. Examples of secondary literature are Index Medicus, International Pharmaceutical Abstracts, and Science Citation Index. "Tertiary literature" refers to those resources which provide overviews of a topic and do not generally contain as much detail as primary or secondary literature. Textbooks are an example of tertiary literature.

3. *Advantages and Disadvantages of Selected Resources*

One of the keys to successfully providing drug information is to know the advantages, disadvantages, and other distinguishing characteristics of the available resources. The accuracy, currency, completeness, and credibility of a response can depend largely on which references were used. Many of the important characteristics of selected resources are described below.

a. Textbooks

Advantages: Textbooks generally provide an overview of a topic and often represent a consensus of opinion, rather than an individual's perspective. Textbooks can be used to quickly review a topic.

Disadvantages: Textbooks often take a long time to be written, edited, and published. Thus, information published in textbooks may quickly become outdated. The age of the information can be assessed by checking the publication date of the textbook and the dates of the references cited in the textbook.

Other characteristics:

Cost: The cost of textbooks can be viewed as either an advantage or a disadvantage, depending on one's perspective and budget. With the cost of some recognized references now exceeding $200, some textbooks are beyond the financial reach of many practitioners and students. However, in comparison to the cost of multiple journal subscriptions or one indexing or abstracting service, a textbook may be a bargain.

Authors: The number and qualifications of authors or contributors to a textbook should be considered. A small number of authors for a very complex, all-encompassing topic may indicate that the authors are writing about topics with which they have little practical familiarity. One would normally expect that it is much more difficult for a few individuals to remain current in a very broad subject area than it is for a larger number of specialists. A large number of authors, however, is not a guarantee of quality in a textbook. Writing styles may vary considerably, resulting in some sections being more current, clear, or detailed than others. The qualifications of the authors (usually listed in the introductory section of the textbook) should also be examined. If the authors appear to serve in a largely administrative capacity, they may be less of an authority on a clinical topic than individuals with an active clinical practice. Conversely, a clinician may have less practical knowledge of administrative topics than an individual whose experience has led to a high-level administrative position.

b.   Journals

Journals contain many types of information: original research articles, review articles, consensus statements, editorials, letters to the editor, corrections or clarifications to previously published material, and advertisements. Characteristics of these types of information will be described below. Considerations in assessing the credibility and potential biases of journals are discussed in Chapter 13.

1)   original research articles

Advantages: Most original research published in journals is subjected to a review by peers of the author(s) or other experts on the topic prior to acceptance for publication. The identity of the authors and the reviewers is generally known only to the journal editorial staff, in order to avoid personal bias. The review process helps to ensure that the conclusions of the study are valid, based on the study design and overall knowledge of the topic. Although the review process and editorial revision do add to the publication lag time (see Disadvantages), original research articles are generally viewed as providing relatively current information at the time they are published (see Chapter 13, Question 2).

Disadvantages: The review and editing of original research articles can result in a lag time between when the study is completed and when it is published. Typical lag times for journals are 6 to 18 months.

By limiting their discussion only to the results discovered in the study, original research papers provide a very narrow view of a topic. Opposing findings may be available elsewhere. One of the purposes of the peer review process is to ensure that the study's findings are placed in perspective with other opinions or findings. However, if the reviewers are not properly selected or rush through their reviews, the research article may not present a balanced view, leaving the reader with a slanted understanding of the topic (see Chapter 13, Question 2).

As described in Section III, many research studies have methodological weaknesses which must be recognized in order to put the validity of the conclusions into perspective.

2)   review articles

Advantages: Review articles often combine the advantages of textbooks and original research articles. They provide an overview of a topic, yet are generally more current than textbooks.

Disadvantages: Like textbooks, review articles basically allow the readers to let another person (the author) draw their conclusions for them. Readers do not have the original data (as could be found in the original research paper) from which to draw their own conclusions.

c.   Indexing and abstracting services

Indexing services provide listings of publications on specific topics. If abstracts are also provided, the reader can get a summary of the article content without having to locate the original paper.

Advantages: Indexing and abstracting services can save considerable time for the searcher by organizing the available literature by topic. Although microfiche or hard copy editions of these services are relatively expensive, they are much less costly than the combined cost of subscriptions to the journals that they cover. On-line versions of these systems can be searched very quickly by experienced searchers, making the search cost quite small relative to the time saved.

Disadvantages: These services use sophisticated indexing systems. Some time investment is usually required to learn the system before it can be easily and quickly used. Because of the cost of the microfiche or hard copy services, or the cost of the computer hardware and software needed to do on-line searching, many individuals in small practice settings consider these services to be too expensive. These services usually do not provide an interpretation of the articles that they index.

When should secondary articles be searched manually and when should they be searched on-line? Knodel and Bierschenk[1] describe several decision factors:

1)   expense

On-line searches involve connect-time charges, royalty fees, and off-line print charges, which vary depending on the database. Start-up acquisition and maintenance costs of hard copies versus computer equipment must also be considered.

2)   time

On-line searching may provide more rapid access to needed literature than manual searching. The lag time between publication of information and its appearance in an on-line database may be shorter than the lagtime for a printed source.

3) results of manual searching

On-line searching may be done to confirm or augment the findings of a manual search.

4) nature of information requests

Topics of media interest may warrant comprehensive searches. Information available in popular literature, rather than traditional medical literature, may be accessed through appropriate on-line databases even though not physically in the medical library holdings.

5) indexing and terminology

Expanded vocabularies and the ability to combine search terms provide advantages for on-line searching.

6) staffing and education

At times, the decision to do a manual or on-line search may be influenced by the needs of the drug information staff or students to acquire additional experience with either of the techniques.

An important issue is whether on-line literature searching is best done by the "end-user" (clinician who will apply the information found) or a search specialist (often a librarian). Haynes and colleagues evaluated the relevance of articles retrieved by reference librarians, clinicians experienced in on-line searching, and clinicians inexperienced in on-line searching.[2] Not surprisingly, the inexperienced searchers found significantly fewer relevant articles than did reference librarians or experienced users (411 versus 742 and 728, respectively). Inexperienced searchers found a smaller proportion of the total number of relevant citations retrieved by all three groups, and retrieved 50% more irrelevant articles (p <0.001). Despite the better performance of librarians in retrieving articles that were relevant and omitting articles that were irrelevant, the librarians failed to retrieve more than half of the relevant citations that were available (as demonstrated by the retrieval of additional relevant articles by the other searchers). Just over half of the searches done were for management of a "patient problem". Half of these were stated to have affected clinical decisions, in the majority of cases, without a full-text article being viewed. The authors conclude that on-line searching with selected software in a clinical setting is "feasible with brief training and that it is popular with users".

A comparison of the usefulness of MEDLINE searches performed by a drug information pharmacist and by more experienced medical librarians showed no significant difference.[3]

d.   Advertisements prepared by pharmaceutical manufacturers

Advantages: Advertisements generally contain very current information, and, in fact, some begin to suggest information or impending product availability even before FDA approval. An advertisement is a convenient place to locate a "package insert" for a prescription drug, because the manufacturer is required to include the approved labeling information with the advertisement. Information in an advertisement for a prescription drug is supposed to be consistent with the FDA-approved product labeling. Advertisements provide very clear highlights of study findings, often in colorful graphic displays which leave a quick but lasting impression.

Disadvantages: Many advertisements do not contain citations for claims, or the citations are for resources which may be unavailable or difficult to locate ("in-house data" or obscure publications not available in most medical libraries). By design, advertisements contain information which shows the product in the best light, possibly leaving a biased impression. Examination of the original data from which claims are made in an advertisement often leaves the reader with a different impression about the product than would be gained from reading the advertisement alone.

e.   Manufacturers' information (e.g., file cards, "detail pieces")

Manufacturers' information is similar to advertisements in many ways, although the amount of information presented is generally greater than in advertisements.

f.   Manufacturers' representatives

Advantages: These individuals may be able to assist in locating relevant information or experts on a topic. They may have reprints of articles available, saving the time and expense of photocopying. Representatives with strong education or training in the therapeutic area may be quite helpful in identifying the important issues and interpreting conflicting or new information.

Disadvantages: The education and training of pharmaceutical manufacturers' representatives varies considerably. While some are quite knowledgeable and helpful, others are aware of only limited information on their products (generally the more positive information) and know even less about their competitors' products. Their job is to present the best impression possible about their product, a position which tends to result in bias in the information that they provide.

The FDA restricts pharmaceutical manufacturers (including sales representatives) from volunteering information which is not consistent with the FDA-approved labeling (package insert). However, if the information is *requested* by a health care professional, the company may provide information it has which is relevant to the request. Some companies will allow their representatives to discuss information outside of the package insert if it is requested voluntarily, while other companies are concerned that accusations of promotion could be made if the representatives are allowed to discuss these topics. Thus, the companies may decline to provide the information or forward the requests to a department in the company which specifically handles these requests.

g.   Manufacturers' headquarters

Many pharmaceutical manufacturers have departments specifically designated to respond to inquiries from health care professionals. Generally, these departments are part of the medical division of the company, rather than sales or marketing. They are usually staffed by individuals with a health care background (pharmacists, physicians, nurses) who are sensitive to the urgency with which information will be needed. Most may be reached by telephone and/or in writing, and some provide around-the-clock coverage in case of emergencies. The easiest way to identify a contact number for these departments is to refer to the index of manufacturers in the *Physicians' Desk Reference*. The following guidelines are offered for obtaining drug information from a pharmaceutical manufacturer:[4]

- Contact the appropriate person by determining whether the company has a specific drug information department, before providing a detailed question.
- Contact the company by telephone, rather than mail, if a rapid (less than two weeks) response is needed.
- Provide a complete description of the question, including how the information will be used.
- Ask for the name of the person handling the request so that follow-up inquiries may be directed to the same person.
- Provide feedback so that the manufacturer will have additional information which may be useful in responding to future inquires.

Advantages: These departments have access to in-house data which have not been (and may never be) published, and are therefore not generally available to individuals outside the company. Individuals in these departments have far more information immediately available to them than do the sales representatives and can also refer the caller to experts on specific topics, if appropriate. They apply critical standards to scientific literature evaluation and will usually provide written documentation of their responses.

Disadvantages: The turnaround time for written responses from these departments is variable, depending on the workload, amount of information requested, sensitivity of the information (and corresponding extent of review required), and other factors. It is sometimes difficult to locate the appropriate person to respond to a question because of the size of the company, unless the company has a designated drug information department and the person who answers the telephone knows where to refer the call.

h.   Newsletters

Newsletters can be divided into two types: those published for use within a specific health care institution (usually by a drug information center) and those published for national distribution. National newsletters generally share the characteristics of review articles, although they may be much more timely. Institutionally or "locally" published newsletters have some distinctions related to the specifics of the institution or locale.

Advantages: Newsletters published for "local" use (within the institution where the newsletter is published) may contain specific, practical pointers which are relevant for that institution. The information is likely to be current.

Disadvantages: The quality of in-house newsletters varies considerably. Because medical practice, procedures, and patient populations vary between institutions, the conclusions of one institution's newsletter may not be entirely relevant to another institution.

i.   Clinicians

A frequent mistake that occurs when trying to locate requested information is an over-reliance on written information sources and failure to ask a clinician who may have experience in the area. Even if one locates considerable written data, the perspective of an experienced clinician can be invaluable. On the other hand, some clinicians may have strong biases which could skew an otherwise objective analysis of the available data.

j.   National or government experts

National or government organizations such as the Food and Drug Administration (FDA), Centers for Disease Control (CDC), United States Pharmacopeial Convention, Inc. (USP), and Environmental Protection Agency (EPA) can also serve as information resources.

Advantages: Authoritative, excellent on epidemiological problems.

Disadvantages: Bureaucratic, difficult to find the best person to answer the question.

References

1.   Knodel LC, Bierschenk NF. Selective use of on-line literature searching by a drug information service. *Am J Hosp Pharm* 1983;40:257-9.
2.   Haynes RB, McKibbon KA, Walker CJ, Ryan M, Fitzgerald D, Ramsden MF. On-line access to Medline in clinical settings. A study of use and usefulness. *Ann Intern Med* 1990;112:78-84.
3.   Wanke LA, Hewison NS. Comparative usefulness of Medline searches performed by a drug information pharmacist and by medical librarians. *Am J Hosp Pharm* 1988;45:2507-10.
4.   Colvin CL. Understanding the resources and organization of an industry-based drug information service. *Am J Hosp Pharm* 1990;47:1989-90.

Factors for an Effective Response

The time spent researching a question and analyzing information is wasted if the response is not effectively communicated to the requestor. Factors which determine whether a response is effective include the following:

1. *Time Frame for Providing the Response*

   Time frame, the length of time between when the question was asked and when the answer was received or needed, is an important factor for an effective response. The response would be far more effective if the question was answered in time for the information to be considered before a decision about the patient's therapy was made, than if the question was answered after the decision was made.

2. *Length of the Response*

   In the hectic schedules of most health care providers, information is far more likely to be used if it can be understood quickly rather than requiring considerable time to digest. Answers should be as short as possible, while providing sufficient supportive documentation to demonstrate reliability and confidence in the response and consideration of relevant factors, some of which the requestor may not have recognized in the original request.

3. *Information Support*

   The response must be adequately supported by reliable sources of information for the requestor to feel confident accepting it. This requirement is particularly true for subjects in which the requestor has little experience and when the risk of injury or liability is high.

4. *Balance*

   The response should be balanced. That is, it should be neither unfairly positive nor negative. Objectivity is mandatory for credibility.

5. *Oral or Written*

   Different circumstances call for responses in either oral or written form (or occasionally, both). Oral answers are preferred when a speedy answer is needed or when it is important for the requestor to have the opportunity to ask questions or discuss certain points of the case. Written answers are preferred when the response is lengthy (for example, when several references are cited), when there is any question about the requestor's ability to clearly interpret the information, or when a written record of the specific response is needed for legal purposes.

Structure of a Drug Information Response

Whether answered orally or in writing, the overall structure of a drug information response is similar. Oral answers are usually much more brief than written answers, but the basic components of the response are the same:

1. Restatement/summary of the original question

2. Assumptions made by the person responding, if any

   In the absence of specific information, the responder may need to make certain assumptions concerning the patient's age, organ function, etc. These assumptions should be stated in the response, particularly if the answer would be <u>different</u> under other circumstances.

3. Brief summary statement of the response

4. Additional detail concerning the method used to arrive at the response and factors considered in formulating the response

5. References

Anticipation of Follow-up Questions

Helpful drug information providers do more than answer isolated questions; they also anticipate the <u>next</u> questions that will or should be asked, and have answers available for these questions, when possible. For example, if the response to a question about the identity of a foreign drug is that the agent is not available in the prescriber's area, the drug information provider should be prepared to suggest an available alternative, even though the requestor did not originally ask for this information.

Oral Consultation

Most patient-specific information requests are answered orally (either by telephone or in person) because this method is more rapid than preparing a written response. Whenever feasible, face-to-face contact is preferable to telephone contact, because direct personal interaction allows for enhanced communication through the use of eye contact and body expression (e.g., hands waved for emphasis). Face to face contact enables the provider to better determine if the requestor understands and can use the response. Telephone conversations tend to be shorter than face-to-face conversations, which may be either an advantage or a disadvantage, depending on the circumstances.

When attempting to reach the requestor to provide a response or obtain additional information, one should be sensitive to the schedule of the individual, if known. For example, an attending physician whose schedule often includes lunchtime meetings may not appreciate being paged during the meeting. Similarly, surgeons who ordinarily are performing procedures in the morning may prefer being contacted in the afternoon. If some time will be required before an answer can be delivered, it is best to ask requestors what time of day is best to contact them. For individuals with particularly hectic schedules, it may be prudent to ask if there are any other individuals who may also receive the response (e.g., a nurse caring for the patient) so that significant time delays do not occur in transmission of the information.

Written Consultation

Drug information in written form is provided in several ways. Very specific responses may be prepared in reply to specific questions, or more general reviews may be written on topics of interest to a wider audience (e.g., newsletter articles, pharmacy and therapeutics committee reviews). In general, the more specific the question, the more specific the response should be. Appropriate background information should be obtained (as discussed in Chapter 9) to determine the exact question that is being asked, and the potential applications of the response. A data collection form is a useful tool for compiling data consistently (Appendix H). Examples of written consultations that were developed in response to questions appear in Appendix I.

Feedback/Evaluation

In the rapid pace of the health care setting, follow-up on the outcome or impact of drug information responses is often lacking. However, this is a very important step and should be included whenever feasible.

For patient-specific inquiries where a firm answer based on prior data is unavailable, the health care professionals involved may be forced to take a "best guess" approach to managing the patient. In these cases, it is wise to determine the outcome in order to gain valuable information for application to future patients in the same situation. In some cases, publication of results may be warranted so that information can be disseminated to a wide audience.

Evaluation of drug information services is also important to help document the contribution the drug information center is making to patient safety, cost containment, or other aspects of the health care system. Potential methods of evaluation include user surveys; drug utilization evaluations; cost-effectiveness, cost-benefit, or cost-minimization studies; or otherwise monitoring health care professionals' behaviors.

SECTION III   *Scientific Literature Evaluation*

Sections I and II focused on the process and environment in which drug information services are provided to health care practitioners. Section III focuses on the process of scientific literature evaluation: evaluating articles that describe clinical drug trials. Chapter 12 provides an overview of the approach while Chapters 13 through 18 provide in-depth instruction regarding how to critically evaluate the various sections of the article.

In 1981 it was estimated that the biomedical literature expanded at a rate of 6% to 7% per year and will double every 10 to 15 years.[1] The prediction was validated in the past decade by the enormous growth in medical information available to health care practitioners. Unfortunately, the growth was accompanied by a wide variation in research quality.[2-7] While many clinical drug trials are methodologically sound, there are sometimes biases in that which gets reported. The primary bias is the tendency to report only "positive" results and not findings that are "negative". Other biases result from the pressure on scientists to publish, causing some to engage in misleading practices such as making exaggerated claims from their findings, fragmenting their results by reporting in multiple journals, conducting and submitting for publication only those clinical drug trials which can be completed and published easily, or providing incomplete descriptions of trial methods and/or results.[8-12] A more serious problem which, fortunately, occurs rarely, is scientific fraud, where false data are created or conflicting or undesirable results are withheld.[13]

Despite the large number of properly designed clinical drug trials published, the health care practitioner is sometimes faced with results that may be conflicting or contradictory. Such results are not attributed to flaws in trial design but to investigators adhering to strict or rigid standards that limit the extent to which the findings can be extrapolated to typical clinical practice. Thus, the health care practitioner is forced to decide which set of conflicting or contradictory findings is most representative of typical clinical practice even though all the research examined may be considered methodologically sound.[14-16] The need to choose among a variety of conflicting or incomplete results can cause confusion among health care practitioners regarding the optimal drug therapy for a particular disease.[2,17-20]

Categorizing Clinical Drug Trials

Clinical drug trials tend to fall into a variety of basic types, although specific classification schemes vary.[21-23] One classification is based on the drug development process in the United States, which is regulated strictly by the Food and Drug Administration.[22,23] The process is divided into separate stages as described in Table 12-1.

Table 12-1.   The United States Drug Development Process[24-26]

Stage	Description	Duration
Preclinical Trials	Assessment of primary safety and biologic activity. Involves animal and *in vitro* studies.	average = 3.5 years
Phase I Clinical Trial	Determination of initial drug safety, and tolerance, including the safe dosage range. Involves 20 to 100 normal healthy adult volunteers.	average = 1 year
Phase II Clinical Trial	First evaluation of drug efficacy, dose response, and side effects in patients in which the drug is intended. Administered to 100 to 500 fairly homogeneous patients.	2 to 5 years
Phase III Clinical Trial	Verification of drug effectiveness and safety, especially in long term use. Establishment of optimum dosage. Administered to 1000 to 3000 volunteer, relatively heterogeneous patients.	2 to 4 years
Phase IV Clinical Trial	Also known as Postmarketing Surveillance. Intended to obtain more information about the benefits and risks associated with the drug's use in the general population. Performed either prior to or after the release of the drug to the consumer market.	Indefinite

1.   Preclinical Trials

Preclinical trials are conducted at the beginning of the drug development process and involve an initial synthesis of the drug (1-3 years) and long-term animal and *in vitro* testing (2-10 years). The main purpose of preclinical trials is to assess initial drug effects: biological activity, pharmacokinetic profile (e.g., rate and degree of absorption, distribution, metabolism, and excretion) and general toxicological profile. The trial design usually involves screening drugs for activity and assessing the dose-response relationship. Because many preclinical trials are performed on specific animal species, extrapolation of the results to humans may be difficult.

2. Phase I Clinical Trials

Phase I clinical trials represent the first introduction of the new drug into humans. They involve various ranges of drug doses and dose schedules in order to focus on initial drug safety and pharmacokinetics. The primary purpose of Phase I clinical trials is to determine which organs may be most adversely affected by the drug, the preferred route of administration, and a safe dosage range. The sample size ranges from 20 to 100 normal healthy adult volunteers. The actual trial design varies with the type of drug being evaluated but commonly involves the use of escalating single doses or short-term, multiple doses.

3. Phase II Clinical Trials

Phase II clinical trials represent the introduction of the new drug into the population for which it is intended. Their primary purpose is to demonstrate the drug's effectiveness while continuing to learn more about the drug's safety. The research in this phase usually consists of controlled studies on a limited number (100 to 500) of patients completed during a relatively short time period. The Phase II clinical trial period typically lasts from 2 to 5 years. Such trials are sometimes used for identifying drugs with the most potential for use in clinical practice so that the drug could be further developed by the manufacturer. In addition, some research may be conducted to determine the importance of certain side effects attributed to the drug.

4. Phase III Clinical Trials

Phase III clinical trials are an expansion of the drug evaluation to larger numbers of patients (1000 to 3000) for substantially longer time periods (3 to 12 months). The purpose of Phase III research is to demonstrate the safety of the drug during longer time periods and continued drug effectiveness without the development of tolerance. The new drug is usually compared with the currently accepted standard drug treatment in the particular disease and/or a placebo (or best supportive care) if no standard exists. The research in this phase tends to last between 2 and 4 years and consists of the most rigorous and extensive evaluation of the new drug, usually involving large scale, well-controlled, multicenter clinical trials.

5. Phase IV Clinical Trials

Phase IV clinical trials (or postmarketing surveillance) include manufacturer-, government-, or other institution-sponsored research on the drug once it is marketed to consumers. In some cases, Phase IV clinical trials are required by the Food and Drug Administration before the drug is given final approval. The principal purpose for the research at this phase of the drug development process is to obtain a better appreciation of the full benefits and hazards of the drug once it is used in the general population. Information typically gathered in Phase IV clinical trials includes the proper dosing for specific populations of humans such as the elderly, limitations of use in patients with certain pathologies such as renal or hepatic impairment, or the existence or frequency of less frequent, but important, side effects. Although the type of research in Phase IV varies, depending on the needs of the manufacturer, the health care practitioner, and the government, it generally includes additional clinical trials similar to those in Phase III, anecdotal reports of side effects (e.g., published case reports), or long-term epidemiological trials (e.g., retrospective and prospective).

Interpreting Different Types of Drug Research Designs

There are many types of drug research designs used in drug development. The health care practitioner needs to be familiar with the advantages and disadvantages of each design in order to effectively interpret the reported results for use in clinical practice. The typical designs used in drug development are animal studies, case control or cohort studies, anecdotal or spontaneous reporting, and clinical drug trials.

1. Animal Studies

Clinicians typically review research from Phase II or III clinical trials when deciding the most appropriate choice of drug therapy. However, there are usually numerous published studies about the drug that are conducted in animals, especially regarding potential toxicities. The animal studies should be applied cautiously in the clinical setting because many side effects observed in humans may not be manifested in animals and vice versa. Using animal research to predict drug effects in humans may lead to erroneous projections because of species differences in the rate and degree of drug absorption, distribution, metabolism, and excretion.[23,27]

2. Case Control or Cohort Studies

Case control (retrospective) or cohort (prospective) studies are often used in Phase IV clinical trials. Case control or retrospective studies go back in time to determine what characteristics are associated with a particular drug effect, usually a side effect. Thus, patients with a certain disease or set of symptoms (which could be a side effect) are examined to determine whether they were taking the drug under research. For example, case control or retrospective studies were used to research the relationship between estrogen use and endometrial cancer.[27-29]

Cohort or prospective studies differ from case control studies because they typically begin with patients taking the drug under research and follow the patients for an extended period of time to determine if they will develop a possible side effect.[21,30,31] For example, a prospective trial of the drugs used by pregnant women would be useful in learning how drug therapy affects the fetus in the first trimester of pregnancy.[30]

While case control and cohort studies are good techniques for assessing the hazards of drug use in clinical practice, causal relationships are more difficult to establish with this type of design compared with clinical drug trials. Primary reasons for the difficulty are the inability to accurately determine the timing of the drug exposure in relationship to the suspected drug effect and the failure to control for the influence of other possible causative factors (see Chapter 18, Question 21).[28,32]

3. Anecdotal or Spontaneous Reporting

Anecdotal or spontaneous reports (sometimes called case reports) are often used in Phase IV research to identify unexpected or previously undetected side effects. Information generated from the case reports can lead to major changes in the manufacturer's product labeling, including removal of the drug from the market. For example, the diuretic ticrynafen (under the brand name Selacryn®) was identified as causing hepatic failure through case reports and was eventually removed from approved use.[30]

Although clinical drug trials have generally replaced case reports as the source of information about drug efficacy, these reports can be useful in situations where decisions cannot be made based on controlled trials. An example would be an unexpected side effect that could be ultimately redefined as a therapeutic effect if certain dosing and drug monitoring conditions are changed. The value of case reports for identifying drug effectiveness is enhanced if two or more treatments are present, repeated measures are implemented, and sophisticated statistical analysis techniques, such as analysis of variance, are used to determine the significance of the reported data.[33-34]

Despite their value, case reports do not replace clinical drug trials as the main source of data regarding the benefits and hazards of drug therapy. The significant biological variation that exists among humans does not enable the clinician to accurately extrapolate drug outcomes from one or two patients to the general patient population.[22]

4.   Clinical Drug Trials

Pocock defines the clinical drug trial as "any form of planned experiment that involves patients and is designed to elucidate the most appropriate treatment of future patients with a given medical condition."[22] Clinical drug trials are considered to be the most effective tool for the evaluation of drug therapy and are the main topic of discussion for the remainder of this chapter and Chapters 13 through 18.[35,36]

Evaluation of Clinical Drug Trials

Although clinical drug trials have contributed greatly to the effective and safe use of drugs, there are difficulties in the interpretation, feasibility and ethics of these trials.[35-38] Because some of the difficulties reported are due to a lack of adequate understanding of the purpose and design of clinical drug trials, Chapters 13 through 18 are devoted to a discussion of how best to understand and apply this type of research. These chapters are organized by the typical sections of a published article which are described briefly in Table 12-2.

Table 12-2.   Typical Structure of Articles Describing Clinical Drug Trials[22,32]

Section	Description
Title	Brief description of the research conducted
Abstract/Summary	Overview of the research conducted
Introduction	Background information for the trial including results of prior research
Methods	Description of drug research design (e.g., criteria for subject selection and number, dosing information, experimental and control groups, measures of efficacy and safety)
Results and Data Analysis	Analysis of research findings, including discussion of dropouts, discontinuation of drug therapy
Discussion/Conclusion	Interpretation of results, comparison to current standard drug treatment, discussion of future implications of research
References	Evidence that prior research has been considered in designing and interpreting the trials

The consistent structure of the articles enables the health care practitioner to identify important aspects of the trial relatively easily. Nevertheless, an organized approach is needed to identify the comparatively few papers that are most applicable to clinical practice.[1] Many schemes are available which address how a health care practitioner should evaluate the results generated from clinical drug trials.[22,31,32,35,38-40] The evaluation process discussed in this book is a hybrid of most of those efforts and is described comprehensively in Chapters 13 through 18. An overview of the evaluation scheme is shown by the checklist in Figure 12-1. Whenever possible, examples of various clinical drug trials are provided to assist in comprehending the principles discussed. In some cases, examples are provided to demonstrate appropriate or inappropriate research techniques. The latter examples are not meant to criticize the research of others and are often derived from the authors' discussion of the limitations of their research design. Most investigators attempt to develop the best research design possible but are sometimes confronted with methodological problems that cannot be avoided.

Figure 12-1.   Checklist of Questions for Evaluating Clinical Drug Trials

Y/N/NA

Abstract and Introduction

1.   Does the abstract concisely discuss all major aspects of the clinical drug trial?   _____

2.   What procedures does the journal use to ensure that quality articles are published?   _____

3.   Is there any information present which suggests bias in the publication of the article?   _____

4.   Does the literature review provide adequate background information?   _____

5.   Are the objectives or purpose of the clinical drug trial clear, unbiased, specific, consistent and important?   _____

Study Design and Methods: Patients and Research Setting

6.   Were the patients selected by appropriate means?   _____

7.   How closely does the clinical drug trial sample represent the pool of patients who will be treated with the drug in clinical practice?   _____

Study Design and Methods: Use of Experimental Controls

8.   How does the patient selection process control for the potential influence of extraneous factors?   _____

9.   What types of control groups were used to compare the effectiveness of the investigational drug treatment?   _____

10.   Was patient assignment to experimental or control groups appropriate?   _____

11.   Were adequate blinding techniques utilized?   _____

Study Design and Methods: Measurement of Results

12.   What methods were used to ensure the quality of the measures used in the clinical drug trial?   _____

13.   How appropriate were the measures of drug effects?   _____

Results and Data Analysis

14.   Were all protocol deviations reported and managed appropriately?   _____

15.   Were all patient retention and data collection problems reported and controlled in the analysis?   _____

16.   Were descriptive statistics used properly to describe the trial results?   _____

17.   Were figures, graphs, or tables used adequately to present the trial results?   _____

18.   Was the approach described by the investigators appropriate for analyzing possible differences between the experimental and control groups?   _____

19.   Were the results of the significance testing interpreted correctly?   _____

20.   What influence does the number of patients analyzed have on the interpretation of the reported results?   _____

Discussion and Conclusions

21.   Was a causal relationship firmly established between the results reported and the use of the investigational drug?   _____

22.   How clinically important are the reported differences between the experimental and control groups?   _____

23.   Have the investigators established that the reported results can be extrapolated to everyday clinical practice?   _____

Y = yes; N = no; NA = insufficient information available

References

1. Sackett DL. How to read clinical journals: I. Why to read them and how to start reading them critically. *CMA Journal* 1981;124:555-8.
2. Haynes RB, McKibbon KA, Fitzgerald D, Guyatt GH, Walker CJ, Sackett DL. How to keep up with the medical literature. II. Deciding which journals to read regularly. *Ann Intern Med* 1986;105:309-12.
3. Woolf PK. Pressure to publish and fraud in science. *Ann Intern Med* 1986;104:254-6.
4. Thorn MD, Pulliam CC, Symons MJ, Eckel FM. Statistical and research quality of the medical and pharmacy literature. *Am J Hosp Pharm* 1985;42:1077-82.
5. Mosteller F, Gilbert JP, McPeek B. Reporting standards and research strategies. *Controlled Clinical Trials* 1980;1:37-58.
6. Nahata MC. Publishing by pharmacists. *Drug Intell Clin Pharm* 1989;23:809-10.
7. DerSimonian R, Charette LJ, McPeek B, Mosteller F. Reporting on methods in clinical trials. *N Engl J Med* 1982;306:1332-7.
8. Newcombe RG. Towards a reduction in publication bias. *Br Med J* 1987;295:656-9.
9. Angell M. Publish or perish: a proposal. *Ann Intern Med* 1986;104:261-2.
10. Bailer JC. Science, statistics, and deception. *Ann Intern Med* 1986;104:259-60.
11. Huth EJ. Irresponsible authorship and wasteful publication. *Ann Intern Med* 1986;104:257-9.
12. Dickersin K, Min YI, Meinert CL. Factors influencing publication of research results. *JAMA* 1992;267:374-8.
13. Angell M, Relman AS. Fraud in biomedical research: a time for congressional restraint. *N Engl J Med* 1988;318:1462-3.
14. Conner CS. Conflicting data in the literature: a true dilemma. *Drug Intell Clin Pharm* 1986;20:444-5.
15. Horwitz RI. Complexity and contradiction in clinical trial research. *Am J Med* 1987;82:498-510.
16. Klimt CR. Varied acceptance of clinical trial results. *Controlled Clinical Trials* 1989;10:135S-41S.
17. Haynes RB, Sackett DL, Tugwell P. Problems in the handling of clinical and research evidence by medical practitioners. *Arch Intern Med* 1983;143:1971-5.
18. Bennett KJ, Sackett DL, Haynes RB, Neufeld VR, Tugwell P, Roberts R. A controlled trial of teaching critical appraisal of the clinical literature to medical students. *JAMA* 1987;257:2451-4.
19. Brink CJ. Reading with a critical eye. *Am J Hosp Pharm* 1986;43:1697.
20. Clemens JD, Feinstein AR. Calcium carbonate and constipation: a historical review of medical mythopoeia. *Gastroenterology* 1977;72:957-61.
21. Bailer JC, Louis TA, Lavori PW, Polansky M. A classification for biomedical research reports. *N Engl J Med* 1984;311:1482-7.
22. Pocock SJ. Clinical trials: a practical approach. New York: Wiley & Sons, 1983:1-7.
23. Nwangku PU, ed. Concepts and strategies in new drug development. New York: Praeger, 1983:3-83.
24. Nicklas RA. The investigative process for new drugs. *Ann Allergy* 1989;63:598-600.
25. Miller HI, Young FE. New biotechnology as a paradigm of a science-based activist approach. *Arch Intern Med* 1989;149: 655-7.
26. Glaxo Inc. Molecule to market: the drug development process. 1991.

27. Reidenberg MM. Species similarities and differences in drug metabolism. *Hosp Pharm* 1975;10:252-3,6.
28. Miettinen OS. The clinical trial as a paradigm for epidemiologic research. *J Clin Epidemiol* 1989;42:491-6.
29. Sartwell PE. Retrospective studies: a review for the clinician. *Ann Intern Med* 1974;81:381-6.
30. Edlavitch S. Practical perspectives on post-marketing surveillance-phase IV. In Nwangku PU, ed. Concepts and strategies in new drug development. New York: Praeger, 1983:101.
31. Riegelman RK, Hirsch RP. Studying a study and testing a test. 2nd ed. Boston: Little Brown, 1989:9-11.
32. Gehlbach SH. Interpreting the medical literature: a clinician's guide. New York, Macmillan Publishing Company, 1988:1-59.
33. Rochon J. A statistical model for the "n of 1" study. *J Clin Epidemiol* 1990;43:499-508.
34. Guyatt GH, Heyting A, Jaeschke R, Keller J, Adachi JD, Roberts RS. N of 1 randomized trials for investigating new drugs. *Controlled Clinical Trials* 1990;11:88-100.
35. Kramer MS. Scientific challenges in the application of randomized trials. *JAMA* 1984;252:2739-45.
36. Friedman LM, Furberg CD, DeMets DL. Fundamentals of clinical trials. 2nd ed. Littleton, MA:PSG Publishing, 1985:ix.
37. Buck C, Donner A. The design of controlled experiments in the evaluation of non-therapeutic interventions. *J Chron Dis* 1982;35:531-8.
38. Barnes RW. Understanding investigative clinical trials. *J Vasc Surg* 1989;9:609-18.
39. Franks P. Clinical trials. *Fam Med* 1988;20:443-8.
40. Ilersich AL, Arlen RR, Ozolins TR, Einerson TR, Mann JL, Segal HJ. Quality of reporting in clinical pharmacy research. *Am J Pharm Ed* 1990;54:126-31.

Chapter 13   Abstract and Introduction

Checklist Questions

1. Does the abstract concisely discuss all major aspects of the clinical drug trial?

2. What procedures does the journal use to ensure that quality articles are published?

3. Is there any information present which suggests bias in the publication of the article?

4. Does the literature review provide adequate background information?

5. Are the objectives or purpose of the clinical drug trial clear, unbiased, specific, consistent and important?

Discussion

The first and often the only exposure that a health care practitioner gets to a clinical drug trial is the beginning of an article, primarily the abstract or introduction. While the abstract should summarize the major parts of the trial, the introduction ought to provide the rationale for doing the research.

Explanation of Checklist Questions

1. Does the abstract concisely discuss all major aspects of the clinical drug trial?

The abstract has evolved from the old "summary and conclusions" section that was traditionally placed at the end of the article and is intended to provide the busy health care practitioner with a time-saving and easy approach to reviewing a clinical drug trial.[1] The value of the abstract as a quick source of information about a clinical drug trial has become more important with the availability of computerized information searching systems such as MEDLINE. Besides the basic features of the article (e.g., authors, title, journal), most computerized information systems provide brief summaries of the research. These summaries are usually the article's abstract. Thus, it is important that the abstract clearly outlines the article's content.[2]

Abstracts are intended to provide a concise summary of the articles and are usually restricted to between 200 and 400 words. A comprehensive abstract usually includes statements regarding the purpose of the trial, research methodology, results reported, and the author's conclusions based on the findings.[3] While a complete description of the research conducted is important, the traditional abstract tends to focus on reporting the results of the data analysis.

Comprehensive abstracts enable the reader to gain a sense of the article's content. However, abstracts can be misleading because the research methodology and results sometimes cannot be sufficiently explained in the limited space allocated. In addition, abstracts are sometimes skewed by authors' tendency to describe the trial in the best possible manner. Thus, the value of a clinical drug trial should not be based on the abstract alone.[1,3-5]

An example of a traditional abstract format is shown in Figure 13-1. The abstract was published in an article describing a clinical drug trial which compared astemizole, terfenadine or placebo in the treatment of patients with hay fever.[6]

Figure 13-1.   A Double-Blind Comparison of Astemizole, Terfenadine or Placebo in Hay Fever with Special Regard to Onset of Action.[6]

In this double-blind study, 47 patients with hay fever were treated for eight days with either terfenadine 60 mg twice a day, astemizole 10 mg once a day, or placebo.

On the second day of treatment terfenadine was statistically significantly superior to astemizole and placebo according to the ratings of symptomatology, efficacy and individual symptoms. The median onset of symptom alleviation was three hours for terfenadine and two days for astemizole.

On the eighth day both astemizole and terfenadine were statistically more efficacious than placebo, but no significant differences were found between the two drugs. Both drugs were well tolerated.

As indicated in Figure 13-1, a major part of the abstract (about 70%) was devoted to the discussion of the results reported. The remainder was a brief description of the research methodology, which included the number of subjects (47), the type of controls (double-blind), duration of the study (8 days), and the dosages of the drugs to be compared. While the results were discussed in-depth, the authors used vague terms such as "astemizole and terfenadine were more efficacious than placebo" and "both drugs were well tolerated" in describing their results. Neither the purpose of the study (i.e., to compare the therapeutic profiles of astemizole and terfenadine, including onset of action) nor the type of measures used were discussed in the abstract.

The need for more summarized information among health care practitioners has generated a movement to urge journals to publish more structured and complete abstracts. In 1987, the Ad Hoc Working Group for the Critical Appraisal of the Medical Literature suggested dividing the abstract in a series of headings as indicated in Table 13-1.[2]

Table 13-1.   Key Abstract Information[2]

Heading	Description
Objective	The exact question addressed by the article
Design	The basic clinical drug trial design, including duration of follow-up
Setting	The location and the type of care provided
Patients/participants	Number of patients who entered and completed the trial, including how they were selected
Interventions	The essential features of the intervention, including the method of administration and duration of therapy
Measurements/results	Important methods of assessing patients and key results reported
Conclusions	Important, clinically relevant conclusions

A number of prominent pharmacy and medical journals have modified and adopted the structured abstract format.[7] Figures 13-2 and 13-3 illustrate how the modified format was used to describe clinical drug trials published in the *Journal of the American Medical Association* and the *New England Journal of Medicine*, respectively.[8-9]

Figure 13-2.   Sample Abstract 1. Treatment of Streptococcal Endocarditis With a Single Daily Dose of Ceftriaxone Sodium for 4 weeks.[8]

Objective	To evaluate the efficacy and safety of ceftriaxone sodium in the treatment of streptococcal endocarditis.
Design	An open, multicenter, noncomparative study with a follow-up of patients from 4 months to 5 years.
Setting	Internal medicine wards and outpatient clinics of hospitals of various sizes in three European countries.
Patients	Fifty-nine patients with defined criteria for streptococcal endocarditis.
Intervention	Ceftriaxone sodium was administered at a once-daily dose of 2 g for 4 weeks.
Outcome Measures	Clinical outcome and microbiological cure rate.
Results	Among the 59 patients, 55 completed the treatment and were followed up for 4 months to 5 years. No patients showed evidence of relapse. Treatment was completely uneventful in 42 patients (71%). A cardiac valve was replaced in four patients (7%) receiving antimicrobial therapy and in six patients (10%) who had completed antimicrobial therapy. One of the 10 valves taken for culture at surgery was positive, but only for microorganisms that were different from the microorganism isolated before the treatment. The treatment had to be interrupted in four patients because of drug allergy. Other side effects were mild except for two cases of reversible neutropenia. The treatment was easy to administer: 27 patients (46%) had no permanent intravenous catheter at any time, seven patients (12%) had such a catheter for less than 4 days. Twenty-three patients (39%) were discharged from the hospital less than 2 weeks after admission.
Conclusions	Ceftriaxone sodium administered at a once-daily dose of 2 g appears to be an effective and safe treatment of streptococcal endocarditis. In hospitals, this agent may be more convenient to administer than penicillin G with or without aminoglycosides. Some patients may even be treated as outpatients.

Figure 13-3.   Sample Abstract 2. The Timing of Prophylactic Administration of Antibiotics and the Risk of Surgical-Wound Infection.[9]

Background	Randomized, controlled trials have shown that prophylactic antibiotics are effective in preventing surgical-wound infections. However, it is uncertain how the timing of antibiotic administration affects the risk of surgical-wound infection in actual clinical practice.
Methods	We prospectively monitored the timing of antibiotic prophylaxis and studied the occurrence of surgical-wound infections in 2847 patients undergoing elective clean or "clean-contaminated" surgical procedures at a large community hospital. The administration of antibiotics 2 to 24 hours before the surgical incision was defined as early; that during the 3 hours after the incision, as perioperative; and that more than 3 but less than 24 hours after the incision, as postoperative.
Results	Of the 1708 patients who received the prophylactic antibiotics preoperatively, 10 (0.6%) subsequently had surgical-wound infections. Of the 282 patients who received the antibiotics perioperatively, 4 (1.4%) had such infections ($p=0.12$; relative risk as compared with the preoperatively treated group, 2.4; 95 % confidence interval, 0.9 to 7.9). Of 488 patients who received the antibiotics administered early, 14 (3.8 %) had wound infections ($p<0.0001$; relative risk, 6.7; 95% confidence interval, 2.9 to 14.7). Finally, of 369 patients who had antibiotics administered early, 14 (3.8%) had wound infections ($p<0.0001$; relative risk, 6.7; 95% confidence interval, 2.9 to 14.7). Stepwise logistic-regression analysis confirmed that the administration of antibiotics in the preoperative period was associated with the lowest risk of surgical-wound infection.
Conclusions	In surgical practice there is considerable variation in the timing of the prophylactic administration of antibiotics, and administration in the two hours before surgery reduces the risk of wound infections.

2.   *What procedures does the journal use to ensure that quality articles are published?*

Editors of most journals use a systematic process and a predetermined set of criteria to determine which of the articles submitted for publication are actually published. Although some articles are authored by the editorial staff of the journal or solicited from writers not on staff, most journal articles are selected from those voluntarily submitted by independent authors. Thus, a journal's reputation is partially based on the process and the criteria which it uses to select articles for publication. The most important part of that process is the use of a peer review system. Peer review is defined as "the assessment by experts (peers) of the material submitted for publication in scientific and technical periodicals."[10]

The peer review system has evolved in an unsystematic fashion beginning with the occurrence of some casual reviews of articles prior to publication in the middle of the 19th century. By the middle of the 20th century, the peer review system was instituted universally. The universal implementation was needed to handle the large numbers of articles submitted to journals for publication and to meet the demands of an increasingly specialized scientific community.[11]

Although varying by journal, the typical peer review system consists of the journal editor sending manuscripts to one to three "experts" for review and comment on the research methodology and the clinical significance of the findings.[12] The peer reviewers, who are usually anonymous to the article authors, typically make independent recommendations to accept, revise, or reject a manuscript for publication. The journal editor usually examines the reviews and decides the final action for the manuscript, often in consultation with associate editors or the editorial staff. Editors of highly respected journals such as the *New England Journal of Medicine* reject about 60% of the articles submitted.[13]

The peer review system has two general goals: 1) to ensure that methodologically sound research articles are published and 2) to introduce into clinical practice research findings that will have an impact on improving the quality of patient care.[14,15] The process is most effective when it accomplishes the specific objectives listed in Table 13-2.

Table 13-2. Desirable Objectives of a Peer Review System[10]

1. Screens out poorly conceived, designed or executed reports of investigations
2. Ensures proper consideration and recognition of other relevant work
3. Leads to helpful revisions and consequent improvements in the quality of manuscripts reviewed
4. Aids in steering research results to the most appropriate journals
5. Raises the technical quality of the field by improving the training, education and motivation of research scientists
6. Puts a stamp of quality on individual papers as an aid to non-experts who may use the results
7. Improves professional acceptance and approval of journals

Although it is the best method to ensure that scientifically valid and important research findings are published, the peer review system is sometimes limited by the lack of clear standards and criteria for peer reviewers to use when evaluating journal articles. While there appears to be a consensus regarding the recommendation to accept the manuscript for publication, reviewers often disagree on what parts of the manuscript need revision before it is published. Disagreements commonly occur over the quality of the writing, the overall presentation of the research, the appropriateness of the statistical analysis, or the type of references used. In addition, some reviewers submit reviews of poor quality, placing more pressure on the editors to decide whether or not to accept the manuscript.[15-17]

Peer review systems are usually not successful in preventing multiple publication of the same article or narrowed subsets of the same research. Scientific fraud is equally difficult to detect.[10,18,19] It is also possible that the peer review process may restrict the introduction of innovative ideas that could eventually lead to significant improvements in patient care.[15]

Other than through the process of submitting a manuscript to a journal for consideration or acting as a reviewer for a journal, it is difficult to learn much about a journal's peer review policies and procedures. However, one approach is to examine the "instructions to the author" section. For example, *JAMA*, a respected journal published by the American Medical Association (AMA), has the following description of their peer review system: "All submitted manuscripts are reviewed initially by a *JAMA* editor. Those manuscripts with insufficient priority for publication are returned promptly. Other manuscripts are sent to expert consultants for peer review. Peer reviewer identities are kept confidential. Author identities are not kept confidential. . . . All accepted manuscripts become the permanent property of the AMA and may not be published elsewhere without written permission from both the author(s) and the AMA."[20]

3. *Is there any information present which suggests bias in the publication of the article?*

Publication bias is defined as the preference for publishing clinical drug trials that report significant or positive results.[21] It has been suggested that clinical drug trials with small or negative results are less likely to be published than research with statistically or clinically significant outcomes.[10,21,22] If such biases occur often, the scientific literature regarding a particular aspect of drug therapy would be distorted toward reporting of primarily positive results.

Publication bias may occur for a variety of reasons. One possible explanation is that overly critical reviewers and editors cause authors to avoid reporting inconsistent, less interesting, or negative results. Another reason may be due to the use of a relatively small number of subjects which makes the true impact of drug treatments difficult to measure and investigators less willing to publish their research. A third explanation is that agencies that sponsor research are interested primarily in positive outcomes. Finally, trials reporting negative or uninteresting results and with serious methodological flaws may be less likely to be published than those demonstrating positive results with similar flaws.[10,21-25]

Learning about the authors of the trial may be useful in determining the extent that the article is biased toward presenting positive results. Although experienced health care practitioners often become familiar with the background or reputation of the authors through continual reading, the less experienced practitioner can gain a sense of the authors' background based on a variety of factors such as their educational background, their place of employment, or references citing their past work.

An important source of bias is the origin of funding for the clinical drug trial. Funding for clinical drug research typically comes from organizations such as the federal government (e.g., the National Institutes of Health), private foundations (e.g., the American Heart Association), professional organizations (e.g., the American Society of Hospital Pharmacists) or pharmaceutical manufacturers. While most sponsored research is presented fairly, investigators may sometimes feel pressured to compromise methodological standards, report only positive results, or exaggerate their findings in order to ensure additional funding from these organizations.[23,25]

4.   Does the literature review provide adequate background information?

A comprehensive literature review provides an overview of earlier research and describes the rationale for performing the clinical drug trial. In addition, examining the reference list cited in the literature review may assist in establishing the investigators' credibility and serves as an additional source of references for those interested in learning more about a particular topic.[26]

The overview of past research should include a brief discussion of the history of treating the disorder, the relative efficacy of previous drug therapy, and any clinical drug trials which compared the new drug with the existing standard drug treatment. Unfortunately, journal space limitations often cause editors to reduce the relative size of the literature review. Thus, most literature reviews do not provide a complete discussion of the past research although an extensive list of references may be supplied. For example, Table 13-3 shows the type of literature review in a series of articles on the comparative efficacy of a new hypnotic drug, zopiclone.

Table 13-3.   Literature Review of the Clinical Use of Zopiclone[a]

Authors (year)	General Drug Therapy[b]	Zopiclone[c]	Comparative Drug Therapy[d]
Agnoli A, Manna V, Martucci N (1989)[27]	20 (54%)	11 (30%)	6 (16%)
Anderson A (1987)[28]	6 (46%)	7 (54%)	
Elie R, Deschenes JP (1987)[29]	11 (35%)	8 (26%)	12 (39%)
Tamminen T, Hansen PP (1987)[30]	9 (56%)	7 (44%)	
Pull CB, Dreyfus JF, Brun JP (1982)[31]	10 (100%)		
Wickstrom E, Giercksky KE (1980)[32]	27 (100%)		

[a]   The numbers in Table 13-3 refer to the number of lines in the article. No attempt was made to standardize the line length.

[b]   General discussion about past treatment of chronic insomnia.

[c]   Discussion of zopiclone including its therapeutic effectiveness, pharmacodynamic profile, and side effects.

[d]   Description of studies that compare zopiclone with other accepted drug therapy for insomnia (e.g., nitrazepam or flurazepam).

As indicated in Table 13-3, the literature review for this new drug focused primarily on the general drug therapy used in the treatment of insomnia and the past evaluation of zopiclone. The discussion of general drug therapy was more extensive in the earlier studies, probably because little was published regarding zopiclone at that time. Very little, if any, information was given on comparative drug treatment.

Investigators are sometimes selective regarding the references they cite. Research may be cited that was completed by the investigators while the efforts of others are disregarded or minimized. In addition, only references consistent with the investigators' beliefs may be used.

Although the lack of a complete discussion of past research can mislead the health care practitioner, the amount of supportive research can also be misrepresented by the citing of redundant, repetitive, divided, or retracted publications. Redundant articles are publications which contain essentially the same material published in more than one journal. Publication of redundant articles is discouraged by most journals but this effort is difficult to enforce. Repetitive articles are similar to redundant articles in that they involve publishing essentially the same material in more than one type of publication. The major difference is that repetitive articles involve material published more often and in a variety of sources such as original research articles, book chapters, abstracts or review articles. Divided articles involve splitting the findings of a single research project into a string of publications. While this practice may be appropriate in some cases, the effort sometimes is solely to lengthen the investigator's publication record.[18,33]

Rarely, articles are later retracted because of innocent research errors or, in most cases, because the research is based on fraudulent data or ideas. Unfortunately, retracted articles often continue to be cited by other investigators. An investigation by Pfeifer and Snodgrass[34] identified 82 retracted studies that were published from 1970 to 1989. These studies were cited an average of nine times after the article was retracted.

Another set of problems in the literature review involves incorrect or imprecise use of the references that are cited by the authors of the clinical drug trial. The problems can be divided into citation errors and quotation errors. Citation errors occur when certain facts about the referenced article are incorrectly listed. These facts include the author's name, article title or the journal source. Major citation errors are often defined as those that prevented a relatively easy and immediate way to identify the source of the reference. Examples of major citation errors include incorrect journal name, omission of the volume or year of the publication, or incorrect page numbers that do not overlap with correct numbers. In contrast, minor citation errors do not prevent location of the citation and consist of incorrect author initials or page numbers of the article. Citation error rates appear to be very high, ranging from 24% to 48%. Major citation errors are reported to occur in approximately 3% to 9% of the references used in publications.[25,35,36]

Quotation errors occur when the original intent of the cited clinical drug trial is inadequately reflected in the literature review. A major quotation error is created if the cited reference either fails to substantiate or even contradicts the statements made in the literature review section. Minor quotation errors do not significantly distort the research findings but tend to oversimplify the conclusions. Quotation errors occur slightly less often than citation errors, with reported incidence rates of 15% to 30%. Major quotation errors reportedly occur in 6% to 27% of the cited references.[26,35,36]

Citation or quotation errors are relatively easy to identify by examining the actual references cited. However, these errors may frustrate the health care practitioner trying to locate the source or may create a negative impression about the investigators' attention to details. Use of misleading or improper references (e.g., redundant, repetitive, divided or retracted publications) is more difficult to detect and can lead the unfamiliar health care practitioner to give more credibility to a statement than it may deserve. The presence of referencing errors creates distrust in the quality of the investigators' preparation for the research by suggesting that references to prior work were not consulted or personally reviewed by the investigators but merely cited or copied from another article.[26]

5. *Are the objectives or purpose of the clinical drug trial clear, unbiased, specific, consistent and important?*

The stated objectives or purpose of a clinical drug trial should clearly describe the trial hypotheses, which are defined as the expected relationships to be measured in the trial or the primary questions that the investigator is most interested in having adequately answered.[4,37] An example of a trial hypothesis or primary question in a clinical drug trial is whether a new cephalosporin will be more effective than other antibiotics when administered to patients suffering from urinary tract infections.

The objectives of the clinical drug trial are usually provided at the end of the introduction section of the article and often consist of one to five concise statements that summarize the research methodology, including the expected outcome of the trial. Evaluation of the objectives involves assessing their clarity, objectivity, specificity, value and consistency with the investigators' conclusions.

Clear objectives often indicate a strong research plan and are easy to evaluate. An example of a clear objective is:

> "The present placebo controlled study compares the hypnotic efficacy and the incidence of following morning residual sequelae [side effects] after the administration of repeated doses of loprazolam and flurazepam in general practice patients suffering from disturbed sleep patterns."[38]

The above objective clearly states what is being planned. The description includes the type of patient being studied, research setting, drugs involved, and drug effects to be measured.

Many clinical drug trials contain more than one objective in order to obtain as much information as possible from the research. Nevertheless, a clinical drug trial should have a clearly defined primary trial objective or it will be difficult for the health care practitioner to determine the main reason why the research was performed. For example, a primary research question may be to assess the therapeutic effectiveness of a new benzodiazepine compared with the current drug therapy for patients with chronic insomnia. Secondary questions could include evaluation of the comparative safety or the relative rates of patient compliance of the two drugs.[37,39]

A clinical drug trial that includes multiple but vaguely connected objectives suggests a poor research methodology because the investigators may be allocating too much attention to achieving their multiple objectives rather than the primary research question.[39] An example of a vaguely connected set of objectives was demonstrated in a clinical drug trial of the effectiveness of a combination product containing trimethoprim and sulfamethoxazole for the treatment of acute bronchitis.[40] The primary objective in this clinical drug trial stated that:

> "Patients treated with trimethoprim and sulfamethoxazole would have a shorter duration of illness as measured by cough, sputum production, fever, and general sense of well-being."

and the secondary objective read:

> ". . . that performing sputum gram stains would allow a more accurate prediction of subjects who would benefit from antibiotic drug therapy."

The secondary objective suggests that the investigators may be too broad in their research plan because it is not closely related to the primary objective. It is also possible that the trial objectives changed during the project, introducing more bias into the reporting of results.

In an attempt to make the health care practitioner's use of published clinical drug trials more efficient, the trial objectives should be reviewed prior to reading the article in order to determine whether the research question asked is of interest.[1,37] The clinical drug trial should be ignored if the objective appears to focus on providing marginally useful information for the standard drug treatment of the illness.[1]

References

1. Sackett DL. How to read clinical journals: I. Why to read them and how to start reading them critically. *CMA Journal* 1981;124:555-8.
2. Ad Hoc Working Group for Critical Appraisal of the Medical Literature. A proposal for more informative abstracts of clinical articles. *Ann Intern Med* 1987;106:598-604.
3. Cuddy PG, Elenbaas RM, Elenbaas JK. Evaluating the medical literature. Part I: abstract, introduction, methods. *Ann Emerg Med* 1983;12:549-55.
4. Friedman LM, Furberg CD, DeMets DL. Fundamentals of Clinical Trials. Littleton, MA:PSG Publishing, 1985: 11, 236.
5. Gehlbach SH. Interpreting the medical literature: a clinician's guide. Lexington, MA:DC Heath and Company, 1982:6-8.
6. Girard JP, Sommacal-Schopf D, Bibliardi P, Henauer SA. Double-blind comparison of astemizole, terfenadine and placebo in hay fever with special regard to onset of action. *J Int Med Res* 1985;13:102-8.
7. Rennie D, Glass RM. Structuring abstracts to make them more informative. *JAMA* 1991;266:116-7.

8. Francioli P, Etienne J, Hoigne R, Thys J, Gerber A. Treatment of streptococcal endocarditis with a single daily dose of ceftriaxone sodium for 4 weeks. *JAMA* 1992;267:264-7.

9. Classen DC, Evans RS, Pestotnik SL, Horn SD, Menlove RL, Burke JP. The timing of prophylactic administration of antibiotics and the risk of surgical-wound infection. *N Engl J Med* 1992;326:281-6.

10. Bailar JC, Patterson K. Journal peer review: the need for a research agenda. *N Engl J Med* 1985;312:654-7.

11. Burnham JC. The evolution of editorial peer review. *JAMA* 1990;263:1323-9.

12. Morgan PP. Author, editor and reviewer: how manuscripts become journal articles. *CMA Journal* 1981;124:664-6.

13. Weller AC. Editorial peer review in U.S. medical journals. *JAMA* 1990;263:1344-7.

14. Cantekin EI, McGuire TW, Potter RL. Biomedical information, peer review, and conflict of interest as they influence public health. *JAMA* 1990;263:1427-30.

15. Horrobin DF. The philosophical basis of peer review and the suppression of innovation. *JAMA* 1990;263:1438-41.

16. Garfunkel JM, Ulshen MH, Hamrick HJ, Lawson EE. Problems identified by secondary review of accepted manuscripts. *JAMA* 1990;263:1369-71.

17. Stossel TP. Reviewer status and review quality: experience of the journal of clinical investigation. *N Engl J Med* 1985;312:658-60.

18. Angell M, Relman AS. Redundant publication. *N Engl J Med* 1989;320:1212-4.

19. Angell M, Relman AS. How good is peer review? *N Engl J Med* 1989;321:827-9.

20. Anon. Instruction to authors. *JAMA* 1993;270:33-9.

21. Newcombe RG. Towards a reduction in publication bias. *Br Med J* 1987;295:656-9.

22. Angell M. Publish or perish: a proposal. *Ann Intern Med* 1986;104:261-2.

23. Hillman AJ, Eisenberg JM, Pauly MV, et al. Avoiding bias in the conduct and reporting of cost-effectiveness research sponsored by pharmaceutical companies. *N Engl J Med* 1991;324:1362-5.

24. Dickersin K, Min Y, Meinert CL. Factors influencing publication of research results. *JAMA* 1992;267:374-8.

25. Pocock SJ. Clinical trials: a practical approach. New York: Wiley & Sons, 1983:240.

26. Neihouse PF, Priske SC. Quotation accuracy in review articles. *Drug Intell Clin Pharm* 1989;23:594-6.

27. Agnoli A, Manna V, Martucci N. Double-blind study on the hypnotic and antianxiety effects of zopiclone compared with nitrazepam in the effective treatment of insomnia. *Int J Clin Pharm Res* 1989;10:277-81.

28. Anderson AA. Zopiclone and nitrazepam: a multicenter placebo controlled comparative study of efficacy and tolerance in insomniac patients in general practice. *Sleep* 1987;10 (suppl 1):54-62.

29. Elie R, Deschenes JP. Efficacy and tolerance of zopiclone in insomniac geriatric patients. *Int Pharmacopsych* 1982;17(suppl 2):179-87.

30. Tamminen T, Hansen PP. Chronic administration of zopiclone and nitrazepam in the treatment of insomnia. *Sleep* 1987;10 (suppl 1):63-72.

31. Pull CB, Dreyfus JF, Brun JP. Comparison of nitrazepam and zopiclone in psychiatric patients. *Int Pharmacopsych* 1982;17(suppl 2):205-9.

32. Wickstrom E, Giercksky KE. Comparative study of zopiclone, a novel hypnotic and three benzodiazepines. *Eur J Clin Pharmacol* 1980;17:93-9.

33. Huth EJ. Irresponsible authorship and wasteful publication. *Ann Intern Med* 1986;104:257-9.

34. Pfeifer MP, Snodgrass GL. The continued use of retracted, invalid scientific literature. *JAMA* 1990;263:1420-3.

35. Eichorn P, Yankauer A. Do authors check their references? A survey of accuracy of references in three public health journals. *Am J Public Health* 1987;77:1011-2.

36. Evans JT, Nadjari HI, Burchell SA. Quotational and reference accuracy in surgical journals. *JAMA* 1990;263:1353-4.

37. Campbell MJ, Machen D. Medical statistics: a common sense approach. Chichester, England: John Wiley & Sons 1990:7-8,63.

38. Murphy JE, Ankier SI. A comparison of the hypnotic activity of loprazolam, flurazepam, and placebo. *Brit J Clin Pract* 1984;(April):141-8.

39. Weintraub M. How to critically assess clinical drug trials. *Drug Ther* 1982;(July):131-48.

40. Franks P, Gleiner JA. The treatment of acute bronchitis with trimethoprim and sulfamethoxazole. *J Fam Prac* 1984;19:185-90.

Checklist Questions

6.   Were the patients selected by appropriate means?

*7.   How closely does the clinical drug trial sample represent the pool of patients who will be
treated with the drug in clinical practice?*

Discussion

An important part of assessing the value of a clinical drug trial involves extrapolating the
reported results to the clinical practice setting. Poor extrapolation of the data often occurs
because the health care practitioner fails to adequately consider differences between the trial
participants and the patients who will actually receive the drug in clinical practice. Differences
between these populations may occur in prominent characteristics such as age, gender, race,
concurrent diseases or changes in end-organ functions (e.g., kidney or liver function).
Dissimilarities may also occur in less obvious factors such as location or setting, patient
willingness to participate, or drug therapy under research.[1-5]

Explanation of Checklist Questions

6.   Were the patients selected by appropriate means?

The typical patient enrollment process for clinical drug trials is shown in Figure 14-1.[6] As
indicated in the figure, the enrollment process begins by identifying the total pool of patients
who would benefit from the drug therapy. This pool is usually called the patient population
(i.e., the entire group of people) suffering from the disease for which the investigational drug
is indicated. A much smaller sample from this population is selected in order to later estimate
how the drug would act when used in clinical practice.[7] The characteristics of this sample are
dependent on a number of factors such as the selection criteria, the quality of the patient
enrollment process, or the number of patients excluded.[2]

Figure 14-1.   Typical Patient Enrollment Process For Clinical Drug Trials[a]

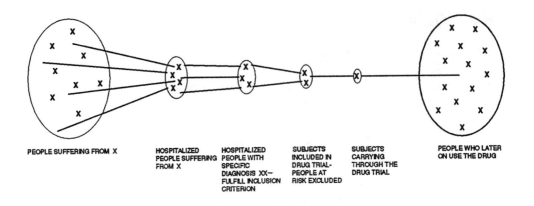

| PEOPLE SUFFERING FROM X | HOSPITALIZED PEOPLE SUFFERING FROM X | HOSPITALIZED PEOPLE WITH SPECIFIC DIAGNOSIS XX— FULFILL INCLUSION CRITERION | SUBJECTS INCLUDED IN DRUG TRIAL- PEOPLE AT RISK EXCLUDED | SUBJECTS CARRYING THROUGH THE DRUG TRIAL | PEOPLE WHO LATER ON USE THE DRUG |

[a]   Adapted with permission from Hansen EH, Launso L. Development, use and evaluation of drugs: the dominating technology in the health care system. *Soc Sci Med* 1987;25:65-73.

a.   Selection criteria

Whenever a clinical drug trial is planned, the existing information about the investigational drug is used to define which patients should or should not receive the drug in the clinical trial (inclusion and exclusion criteria). Inclusion criteria are the requirements which must be met for a patient to be eligible for the trial, and usually consist of characteristics such as age, gender, race, medical condition, or other features such as medical setting and drug therapy. Exclusion criteria are often not explicitly stated but describe characteristics which make a patient ineligible to participate in the clinical drug trial. Those patients typically excluded from a trial are atypical of the population for whom the investigational drug was intended, less likely to benefit from the therapy, or have confounding conditions (e.g., kidney disease) which make establishing drug efficacy and safety difficult.[2]

Selection criteria should be as broad as possible to ensure adequate patient enrollment and extrapolation, but narrow enough to exclude those who may be harmed or who are unlikely to benefit from the drug therapy.[8] Broad selection criteria simplify the screening process, increase the likelihood of meeting enrollment goals and obtaining a large sample size, and improve the applicability of the results. However, narrower selection criteria are important because they increase the likelihood of achieving statistically meaningful results or enable the investigators to more effectively target patients who are most suitable for the drug therapy under research.[9]

The prerequisites for selecting patients often vary significantly among clinical drug trials, primarily due to the differing backgrounds, experience, and philosophy of the investigators.[9] Nevertheless, the criteria used to select patients for a clinical drug trial should be expressed in clear, unambiguous terms. Clear inclusion criteria were illustrated in a clinical drug trial that compared the efficacy and safety of four nonsteroidal anti-inflammatory drugs (ibuprofen, fenoprofen, naproxen, and tolmetin) in the treatment of rheumatoid arthritis. The inclusion criteria consisted of satisfying the American Rheumatism Association diagnostic guidelines for either classical or definite rheumatoid arthritis, having active rheumatoid disease for at least five months after its first articular manifestation, and being a consenting adult receiving care at one of the trial sites.[10]

Clear exclusion criteria were shown in a clinical drug trial that examined the efficacy and safety of low-dose, weekly oral methotrexate therapy for the treatment of inflammatory arthritis. Patients were excluded from the trial if they had abnormal kidney or liver function, as defined by the investigators. These selection criteria were used because of the high potential for dangerous accumulation of the drug in the body or variable efficacy caused by altered drug elimination. Patients were also excluded if they could be treated effectively with less toxic agents (e.g., gold, penicillamine or hydroxychloroquine therapy).[11]

b.   Quality of the patient enrollment process

The patient enrollment process describes how patients were recruited and selected to participate in the clinical drug trial. Successful patient enrollment can be difficult and is dependent upon the type of medical condition under research and the size of the potential pool of patients. A properly designed clinical drug trial should always have a comprehensive process for enrolling patients.[2,12,13] The typical enrollment process begins when patients or their physician perceive a need for drug treatment. Patients may be enrolled in the clinical drug trial if they meet the inclusion criteria, if their physician is willing to participate and to abide by the clinical drug trial protocols and procedures, and the patient formally consents to be entered into the trial. Once enrolled, the patient is assigned to a treatment group and must agree to assist or participate in the completion of all research forms.[4]   Because of the complexity of the patient enrollment process, investigators rarely report meeting their enrollment goals.[13,14,15]

The ideal method of selecting patients for participation in a clinical drug trial is through random choice of patients from the pool of individuals who would likely receive the drug in the clinical setting. In a random enrollment process, each member of the trial population has an equal or known chance of being selected.[16] Thus, randomly chosen trial participants are more likely to be considered representative of the patients who would ultimately benefit from using the drug. Unfortunately, trial patients are rarely randomly chosen because of the unavailability of large pools of eligible individuals. The more common approach is to select eligible patients that either arrive consecutively at a research site or who are referred to the trial by a participating physician. This nonrandom enrollment process is sometimes called a "convenience" sample and is dependent on the bias or preferences of the individual who selects the patients.[2]

An important source of bias in a nonrandom enrollment process is the participating physician. In the treatment of cancer, for example, physician bias toward a particular drug treatment may play an important role in who gets selected to participate in the clinical drug trials for that set of diseases.[17] Reasons why physicians avoid certain patients were examined in a large, multicenter clinical drug trial on breast cancer. The most common reasons were concern about negative effects on the doctor-patient relationship, difficulty with the informed consent procedure, uncertainty of investigational treatment, and conflict with the scientific requirements of the trial versus the clinical need to serve the patient.[18]

c.   Reporting of patients who were excluded

Because published clinical drug trials rarely describe the patients who were excluded from the trial, it is difficult to determine the number of potential participants who were eliminated during the enrollment process. The number is likely to be very high based on the review of Charlson and Horwitz of 41 clinical drug trials, which indicated that only 34% achieved their projected enrollment figures, primarily due to patient or physician refusals.[14] Hunninghake and colleagues[15] estimated that exclusion criteria and patient unwillingness to participate in a clinical drug trial can reduce the enrolled number of participants to less than 10% of the expected number, particularly in large scale multicenter clinical drug trials. The result of poor enrollment of eligible participants is an overrepresentation of certain types of individuals including patients who are Caucasian, married, or those who achieved higher educational levels compared with nonparticipants (see Chapter 17, Question 15).[15,19-21]

7.   *How closely does the clinical drug trial sample represent the pool of patients who will be treated with the drug in clinical practice?*

Regardless of the process used, the individuals enrolled in the clinical drug trial should be compared with the larger pool of patients who are expected to ultimately benefit from the investigational drug in order to determine how representative the reported trial results will be. The representativeness of a sample can be assessed by examining key characteristics of the patients enrolled in the clinical drug trial. Some of these key characteristics are listed in Table 14-1 and need to be described in the trial in order to make the best assessment of the similarity between the trial patients and those who will be using the investigational drug in clinical practice.[3]

Table 14-1.   Representativeness of the Trial Sample: Characteristics for Assessment

Characteristic	Example
Patient demographics	age, gender, race
Medical condition	clear diagnosis
Medical setting	hospital or academic setting
Drugs used	drug regimen, duration of therapy, route of administration

a.   Patient demographics: age, gender, and race

Often clinical drug trials predominantly admit participants who are young or middle aged white males.[15,19-21]   The reported results of clinical drug trials with these types of participants have limited applicability, particularly for certain age groups such as the elderly.[22] Almost any drug action in the elderly has greater variation than in the younger population, primarily due to differences in organ function, concurrent disease states, and concomitant drug therapy.[21,23]

Women and minorities are two other groups often under represented in clinical drug trials. Women were not represented in a National Institutes of Health (NIH) sponsored clinical drug trial on the use of aspirin in the prevention of acute myocardial infarction even though the disease is a major cause of death in this gender group.[19] The relatively low number of minority patients in NIH-sponsored clinical drug trials for the treatment of cancer may have produced misleading findings in types of cancer where race can influence the course of the disease (e.g., cervical or esophageal cancer, myeloma).[24] The problem of underrepresentation of women and minorities has initiated a recent requirement by the NIH that all research proposals submitted to that organization ensure gender and minority representation consistent with the known incidence/prevalence of the disease under research.[19,25]

b.   Medical condition

The diagnostic procedures used to identify the medical condition of the patient enrolled are rarely described comprehensively in most published clinical drug trials. For example, in a review of 51 trials involving patients with congestive heart failure (CHF), only 23 (45%) specified criteria for the diagnosis of CHF.[26] Even if described clearly, the standards used to diagnose major medical conditions may be ambiguous.[1] The lack of standards creates inconsistency among patient outcome measures, causing difficulty in extrapolating the findings to clinical practice. This problem is illustrated in a review of the research on acute myocardial infarction.[27] The diagnostic techniques used to detect acute myocardial damage have changed greatly since the mid-1960's as a result of the increased sensitivity of laboratory tests and more advanced autopsy techniques. The improved diagnostic process alone may have contributed to the significant decline reported in the rates of the disease from 1960 to 1990.

Extrapolation of investigational drug effects in clinical drug trials of patients with variable medical conditions (such as vasospastic angina, rheumatoid arthritis, congestive heart failure, and renal stones) is a problem if the patients are suffering from the condition in its most severe phase when they are enrolled in the trial. Based on a statistical phenomenon known as regression to the mean, the patients selected are likely to improve when measured a second time even if other factors remain constant. Regression to the mean is defined as a set of unusual or rare values with a low probability of recurrence. Thus, any drug treatment will appear to lessen disease activity even though the change may be due to the natural improvement of the illness.[28]

Although most clinical drug trials focus on enrolling patients with a diagnosed form of the disease targeted, some participants are entered into the trial based on their relatively better health compared with the patients who suffer from the medical condition. These individuals tend to be workers, volunteers, or personnel from an organization which typically encourages its members to participate in drug research (e.g., the armed forces or the penal system).[22,29,30] While healthy volunteers may be similar in many ways to the larger pool of patients who will eventually receive the drug, the great proportion are likely to not be completely representative. Even the use of healthy volunteers for drug toxicity studies can be misleading. In a trial of 398 healthy volunteers not receiving any medication, the investigators noted that 13% of the sample reported some symptom that could be attributed to an adverse drug reaction. The most common symptoms were headache, cold-like signs, or backache.[31]

c. Medical setting

Many study participants are recruited from academic research centers or hospital settings because these locations are more likely to include experienced investigators and are better able to skillfully handle new treatment procedures. Unfortunately, the patients who visit these settings tend to have advanced forms of the disease under research. Thus, the patients may respond differently to the investigational drug than individuals who typically use the drug in clinical practice.[4,6]

d. Drugs used: drug regimen, route of administration, duration of therapy

The method in which drugs are used in a clinical drug trial may vary significantly from their use in clinical practice. Differences may occur in the route of administration, the drug dose and schedule, and the duration of therapy.[4,32,33] The route of administration typically differs when products are expected to be used in both the hospital and ambulatory care setting. Drugs under research in the hospital setting may be administered intravenously to more severely ill patients while in the ambulatory care setting the drugs may be administered orally or subcutaneously to less ill patients.

The drug dose and schedule used in many clinical drug trials are often based on the requirements of the drug development process. The amount and frequency of the drug doses are usually determined in Phase I or II clinical drug trials (see Chapter 12 for a description of these type of trials) where the objective is to give the highest effective drug dose that will not cause serious side effects. These trials are sometimes called dose ranging studies. Higher doses are often required to avoid undertreatment or the ethical problem of administering subtherapeutic doses, especially for certain conditions such as severe infections.[4,32,34,35] Unfortunately, the dosing schedules used in drug development are sometimes too rigid and not based on uniform dose-ranging techniques.[4,34,36] Thus, the total amount of the drug given during the drug development process may be too high for the patients in the clinical practice setting (resulting in increased toxicity) or too low (causing a suboptimal therapeutic effect).

Duration of therapy should be considered in assessing the representativeness of the investigational drug therapy from a clinical drug trial.[4] Drugs administered for the treatment of acute conditions such as urinary tract infection are usually evaluated for a time period equivalent to the recommended duration of therapy in clinical practice. However, determining an appropriate time period for clinical evaluation of drugs administered in the long-term treatment of chronic diseases is more difficult because of the expense of performing long-term clinical drug trials, the regulatory requirements of the Food and Drug Administration, and the inherent methodological problem of measuring clinical response over an extended period of time. Thus, there is wide variation in how different investigators define the accepted length of investigational drug therapy for the trial. The variation can have negative consequences if the duration chosen is not suitable to thoroughly assess the investigational drug effect, particularly the less common side effects.[2]

References

1. Riegelman RK, Hirsch RP. Studying a study and testing a test. 2nd ed. Boston: Little Brown, 1989:60-4, 147-9.
2. Friedman LM, Furberg CD, DeMets DL. Fundamentals of clinical trials. 2nd ed. Littleton, MA:PSG Publishing, 1985:23-30, 152.
3. Sackett DL. How to read clinical journals. I. Why to read them and how to start reading them critically. *CMA Journal* 1981;124:555-8.
4. Pocock SJ. Clinical trials: a practical approach. New York: Wiley & Sons, 1983:34-41;66-8;176-9.
5. O'Connell JB, Mason JW. The applicability of results of streamlined trials to clinical practice: the myocarditis treatment trial. *Stat Med* 1990;9:193-7.
6. Hansen EH, Launso L. Development, use and evaluation of drugs: the dominating technology in the health care system. *Soc Sci Med* 1987;25:65-73.
7. Campbell MJ, Machen D. Medical statistics: a common sense approach. Chichester, England: John Wiley & Sons, 1990:54.
8. Franks P. Clinical trials. *Fam Med* 1988;20:443-8.
9. Yusuf S, Held P, Teo KK. Selection of patients for randomized controlled trials: implications of wide or narrow eligibility criteria. *Stat Med* 1990;9:73-86.

10. Gall EP, Caperton EM, McComb JE, et al. Clinical comparison of ibuprofen, fenoprofen calcium, naproxen and tolmetin sodium. *J Rheumatol* 1982;9:402-7.
11. Boh LE, Schuna AA, Pitterle ME, Adams EM, Sundstrom WR. Low-dose weekly oral methotrexate therapy for inflammatory arthritis. *Clin Pharm* 1986;5:503-8.
12. Nwangku PU, ed. Concepts and strategies in new drug development. New York: Praeger, 1983:101.
13. Prout TE. Patient recruitment: other examples of recruitment problems and solutions. *Clin Pharmacol Ther* 1979;25:695-6.
14. Charlson ME, Horwitz RI. Applying results of randomized trials to clinical practice: impact of losses before randomization. *Br Med J* 1984;289:1281-4.
15. Hunninghake DB, Darby CA, Probstfield JL. Recruitment experience in clinical trials: Literature summary and annotated bibliography. *Controlled Clinical Trials* 1987;8(suppl):6S-15S.
16. McAuley WJ. Applied research in gerontology. New York: Van Nostrand-Reinhold, 1987:130.
17. Ganz PA. Clinical trials: concerns of the patient and the public. *Cancer* 1990;65:2394-9.
18. Taylor KM, Margolese RG, Soskolne CL. Physicians' reasons for not entering eligible patients in a randomized clinical trial of surgery for breast cancer. *N Engl J Med* 1984;310:1363-7.
19. Rehm D. Is there gender bias in drug testing? *FDA Consumer* 1991;(April):9-13.
20. Svensson CK. Representation of American blacks in clinical trials of new drugs. *JAMA* 1989;261:263-5.
21. Kitler ME. The changing face of clinical trials. *J Hypertension* 1988;6(suppl 1):S73-S80.
22. Svensson CK. Ethical considerations in the conduct of clinical pharmacokinetic studies. *Clin Pharmacokinet* 1989;17:217-22.
23. Bell JA, May FE, Stewart RB. Clinical research in the elderly: ethical and methodological considerations. *Drug Intell Clin Pharm* 1987;21:1002-7.
24. Friedman MA, Cain DF. National cancer institute sponsored cooperative clinical trials. *Cancer* 1990;65(suppl):2376-82.
25. Anonymous. NIH/ADAMHA policy concerning inclusion of women in study populations. *NIH Guide* 1990;19:17-9.
26. Marantz PR, Alderman MH, Tobin JN. Diagnostic heterogeneity in clinical trials for congestive heart failure. *Ann Intern Med* 1988;109:55-61.
27. Burke GL, Edlavitch SA, Crow RS. The effects of diagnostic criteria on trends in coronary heart disease morbidity: the Minnesota Heart Survey. *J Clin Epidemiol* 1989;42:17-24.
28. Spector R, Park GD. Regression to the mean: a potential source of error in clinical pharmacological studies. *Drug Intell Clin Pharm* 1985;19:916-9.
29. Sterling TD, Weinkam JJ, Weinkam JL. The sick person effect. *J Clin Epidemiol* 1990;43:141-51.
30. Amori G, Lenox RH. Do volunteer subjects bias clinical trials? *J Clin Psychopharmacol* 1989;9:321-7.
31. Kulkarni RD, Vakil BJ. Baseline spontaneous symptoms in healthy persons-a prospective study. *J Clin Pharmacol* 1975;15:442-5.
32. Finkel M. in: Nwangku PU, ed. Concepts and strategies in new drug development. New York: Praeger, 1983:17-22.
33. Weintraub M. How to critically assess clinical drug trials. *Drug Ther* 1982;(July):131-148.

34. Polk RE, Hepler CD. Controversies in antimicrobial therapy: critical analysis of clinical trials. *Am J Hosp Pharm* 1986;43:630-40.
35. Sheiner LB, Beal SL, Sambol NC. Study designs for dose-ranging. *Clin Pharmacol Ther* 1989;46:63-77.
36. Chiou WL. Discrepancies in recommended dosage regimens of drugs. *J Clin Pharmacol* 1976;16:6-7.

Checklist Questions

8. *How does the patient selection process control for the potential influence of extraneous factors?*

9. *What types of control groups were used to compare the effectiveness of the investigational drug treatment?*

10. *Was patient assignment to experimental or control groups appropriate?*

11. *Were adequate blinding techniques utilized?*

Discussion

Investigators of clinical drug trials attempt to prove a causal relationship between the introduction of the investigational drug and the subsequent effect measured. This objective is usually accomplished by comparing the experience of one group of patients who receive the investigational drug (the experimental group) with a group of patients having the same condition who are not receiving identical drug treatment (the control group). Generally, if the subsequent state of illness in the experimental group has improved relative to the control group, the investigational drug treatment is considered to be more effective.[1-3]

The conclusion that the investigational drug treatment is better, equal, or less effective than the drug treatment administered to the control group is based on the investigator's ability to minimize the effect of other factors besides the drug on the patient's therapeutic outcome.[4] A common factor is the possibility that the patient's illness may have simply run its course and recovery would have occurred with no treatment. Another factor is the successful guessing by the clinician or the patient of the expected effects of the investigational drug treatment which may influence the interpretation of the drug's effectiveness. A third factor is the possibility that the patients in the experimental and control groups may be sufficiently unequal to present different responses to the drug treatment. Investigators designing clinical drug trials must control as many of these extraneous factors as possible in order to ensure that the investigational drug treatment was primarily responsible for the effects reported.[1,3]

The basic outline of methods to control the influence of potential extraneous factors is demonstrated in Figure 15-1 and described by Polk and Hepler.[2]

Figure 15-1.   Basic Design for Controlled Clinical Drug Trials

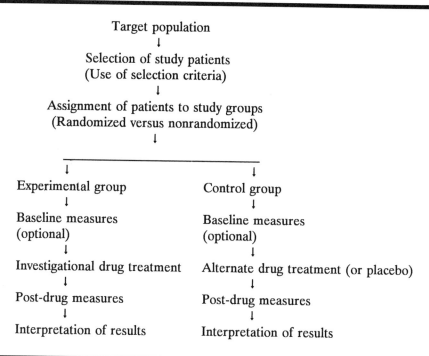

Target population
↓
Selection of study patients
(Use of selection criteria)
↓
Assignment of patients to study groups
(Randomized versus nonrandomized)
↓

Experimental group	Control group
↓	↓
Baseline measures (optional)	Baseline measures (optional)
↓	↓
Investigational drug treatment	Alternate drug treatment (or placebo)
↓	↓
Post-drug measures	Post-drug measures
↓	↓
Interpretation of results	Interpretation of results

One limited method of control is the restriction of potential interfering factors through the use of narrow selection criteria. Another more effective approach is the use of experimental and control groups. A number of possible control groups can be used, depending on the drug being tested or the disease under research. The most typical approach is the use of a parallel control group in which two or more groups are treated separately but concurrently as part of the same clinical drug trial. Another method uses patients as their own controls through the crossover design in which the participants receive both the test and control treatments during separate and specified periods of time. A less frequent approach is the use of historical controls in which the experimental group is compared to previous groups of patients not enrolled in the present trial.[5-6]

Once the appropriate experimental and control group is selected, the investigator needs to ensure that the groups are equal in everything except the drug treatment that will be administered. The ideal method is the random assignment or allocation of patients to each group. The investigator also needs to consider the use of blinding techniques, which reduce the likelihood that investigators or patients can influence the trial results through their preferences or inclinations toward a specific outcome.[1,2,7]

Explanation of Checklist Questions

8. *How does the patient selection process control for the potential influence of extraneous factors?*

Patient selection controls are defined as those techniques used in the selection process which can reduce the influence of extraneous patient-related factors, other than the investigational drug, on the trial results. The most important technique is the use of narrow patient selection criteria. For example, patients are often excluded from a trial if they have diseases other than the condition being studied or are taking drugs other than the investigational drug. While this selection technique makes the groups more similar to each other, it also reduces the extent in which the results can be extrapolated to clinical practice (see Chapter 14).[2,8-9]

9. *What types of control groups were used to compare the effectiveness of the investigational drug treatment?*

Although no standardized categorization exists, the types of control groups used in a clinical drug trial may be divided into three major categories: parallel, crossover and historical controls.[5] The most common type are parallel control groups.

  a. Parallel control groups

The purpose of parallel control groups is to compare the relative effects of different drugs or treatments on two or more groups treated separately but concurrently.[5-6] While the experimental group receives the new drug, the control group could receive a variety of other treatments: a standard drug treatment, a placebo, or no drug at all. The basic design for parallel control groups is similar to the approach in Figure 15-1.

The most common form of parallel control groups is the use of the "standard" drug treatment for the disease under research. This type of control is sometimes referred to as "active control treatment". The objective of using standard drug treatment as controls is to demonstrate that the investigational drug is superior or equivalent in efficacy and safety to the most commonly used drug therapy. One example would be the comparison of a new platelet anti-aggregating agent, ticlopidine, with aspirin for the prevention of stroke. Another example is the use of low dose versus standard dose zidovudine (AZT) treatment for patients with acquired immunodeficiency syndrome (AIDS) or advanced AIDS-related complex.[10]

The goals of clinical drug trials using standard drug treatment controls can be compromised by the type of standard drug treatment used. It is possible that the standard drug treatment chosen may not be the best alternative available. In the comparison of ticlopidine with aspirin for the prevention of stroke, the choice of aspirin as the standard is questionable because the drug has not been previously established to be unequivocally superior compared with placebo. Thus, although clinical drug trial results demonstrated that ticlopidine was equal in efficacy and safety to aspirin, it was not clear that either drug was very effective in preventing stroke.[10]

A second form of a parallel control group design is the use of placebo alone or in combination with other types of control groups. In this type of control, the placebo is an inactive agent that resembles the investigational or active drug in all characteristics such as appearance, route of administration or dosage schedule. The purpose of giving the placebo is to correct for any psychological effects derived solely from medication-taking or from receiving an injection. The use of placebos improves the likelihood that patients will not alter the reporting of symptoms in an attempt to gratify their physician or the study investigators. In addition, the presence of this type of control group in a clinical drug trial minimizes the influences of the investigator's natural partiality toward the positive effects of the investigational drug treatment (see Question 11). The value of placebo controls was demonstrated in a clinical drug trial of hypertension where the conditions of some patients improved more on placebo, raising questions about the reported effectiveness of the investigational drug.[11,12]

Placebos are very useful as additional controls in clinical drug trials in which standard drug treatment is used. It is often automatically assumed that the standard drug treatment with a past history of effectiveness and safety will be equally efficacious and safe under a new set of trial conditions. Unfortunately, this assumption is not always correct, particularly when the condition under research is highly variable or when the efficacy of the standard drug treatment is not firmly established. Thus, demonstration of the superiority of the standard drug treatment relative to placebo may be very important.[10]

Although ethical reasons make denying drug treatment difficult, control groups receiving no treatment or placebo should be used in clinical drug trials where effective drug treatment is not feasible or available.[1] For example, a treatment group not receiving drug therapy would be useful in a clinical drug trial evaluating the management of the common cold. Because the symptoms of a cold are self-limiting, the investigational drug (e.g., a decongestant) should be compared with a control group who received no drug treatment. However, this type of control would be less useful if information about other possible drug treatments is desirable.[1,13]

Controls consisting of no treatment are difficult to implement in patients suffering from the disease under research unless adequate procedures are established to prevent the patients from taking unrecorded medications that could have effects similar to the investigational drug. These procedures include asking patients to report any additional drugs taken during the trial period, providing the control patients with a recorded number of medications to be used when needed to relieve severe symptoms, or institutionalizing the patient during the trial. [1,13]

b. Crossover control groups

Drug research designs using crossover control groups involve having the same patient receive both the investigational and control drug during separate, specified periods of time (Figure 15-2). The patient's reactions to each drug are compared in order to minimize the influence of individual patient characteristics on the response to treatment.[3,14] Crossover designs need fewer participants because each patient serves as both the investigational and control patient. The success of clinical drug trials using a crossover design is based on a variety of factors: carry over or period effects, treatment sequencing or drug order effects, and patient dropout or other data collection problems.

Figure 15-2.   Basic Design for Clinical Drug Trials Using Crossover Control Groups

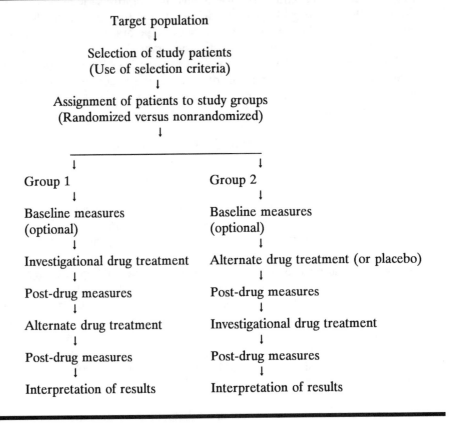

Target population
↓
Selection of study patients
(Use of selection criteria)
↓
Assignment of patients to study groups
(Randomized versus nonrandomized)
↓

↓	↓
Group 1	Group 2
↓	↓
Baseline measures (optional)	Baseline measures (optional)
↓	↓
Investigational drug treatment	Alternate drug treatment (or placebo)
↓	↓
Post-drug measures	Post-drug measures
↓	↓
Alternate drug treatment	Investigational drug treatment
↓	↓
Post-drug measures	Post-drug measures
↓	↓
Interpretation of results	Interpretation of results

1)   carry over effects

Carry over effects occur when the pharmacologic effects of the first or preceding drug treatment persists during the administration of the second or subsequent drug treatment. The common approach to minimizing the influence of these effects is to delay administration of the second or next drug treatment by an appropriate time period, which could be partially based on the drug's pharmacologic half-life (i.e., the amount of time it takes for 50% of the drug to be removed from the body). The time allowed for the delay of the next treatment is commonly called the washout period.

An example of the use of a washout period occurred in a study that compared the inhalant effects of the bronchodilators albuterol, isoetharine and metaproterenol on airway obstruction in 60 adult men.[15] Because the pharmacologic half-lives of these drugs are less than five hours,[16] the investigators chose a 24-hour washout period to ensure that a carry over effect would not occur.

2)   period effects

Period effects appear when the condition under research becomes more severe, less severe or fluctuates in severity during the trial period. For example, drug treatment for a variable disease such as osteoarthritis would be difficult to evaluate using a crossover design because the fluctuations of the symptoms may mask the patient's response to drug therapy. Clinical drug trials containing large numbers of patients may reduce the effect of disease fluctuations because the variability of the disease would be spread evenly across the patients. Nevertheless, results reported from crossover studies in these types of conditions should be interpreted cautiously.

3)   treatment sequencing or drug order effects

Treatment sequencing or drug order effects occur when the sequence of the drug treatment influences the results. An effective method to prevent such influences would be the random assignment of patients to the sequence in which each of the drugs under research will be administered. A rule should also be established prior to the trial indicating when the patients switch to the next drug treatment. The most accepted rule is to automatically switch at a pre-established length of time. A less preferred rule is to switch based on how the condition is progressing.

4)   patient dropout effects

The effects of patient dropout or other data collection problems are more pronounced using crossover control groups compared with parallel control groups because each patient represents a larger proportion of the data collected. Patient dropout rates can be high in crossover studies because patients must receive at least two treatments to provide enough meaningful information for analysis. Patient dropout and other data collection problems are less pronounced in crossover studies that involve short term drug treatment with few severe side effects than in long-term clinical drug trials of more toxic drugs.

5)   N of 1 studies

A derivation of the crossover design is a research scheme in which a single patient is exposed to both the investigational drug and a placebo or an alternative treatment. The method is usually referred to as a "N of 1 study" but has also been labeled a "single case experiment" or "intensive research design." N of 1 studies are different than conventional crossover studies because the focus is on assessing the benefit of drug treatment for an individual patient, not the overall effect on a group of patients. The primary purpose of N of 1 studies is to find the best treatment for a particular patient. Therefore, the results of N of 1 studies should be applied to only the patients who participate in the study.[4]

c.   Historical or external control groups

Drug research designs using parallel control groups or crossover control groups are sometimes called "internal controls" because the patients are enrolled in the control group at about the same time as the patients in the experimental group. "Externally controlled" studies make use of control groups from another time period. These types of controls are also known as historical controls.[7]

Historical control groups can be definitely described or indirectly implied by the investigators. Although some study investigators report no control groups being used, they usually consider some comparison group even though it may be described vaguely as the "existing practice" of using a particular drug treatment or as "no drug treatment." Clinical drug trials using historical controls range from almost casual observations of possibly important relationships to tightly designed exploratory studies such as those used in Phase I clinical drug trials (see Chapter 12).[7]

1)   sources

Two common sources of historical controls are data obtained from the published literature or data already present within the organization.[1,17] Data obtained from the literature consist of information collected from patients treated elsewhere who were previously described in a published report. Such controls usually provide a very poor comparison because it is likely that the experimental group is different than the control group in many aspects other than the drug treatment (e.g., patient selection procedure, experimental environment, and study measures).

Data already present within the organization consist of patient information obtained from the same institution currently conducting the clinical drug trial, but during a previous time period. Although more dependable than data obtained from outside the organization, the reliability of this information is limited because the analysis reported may be too vague to interpret, certain important factors or outcomes may have not been controlled or assessed, or some experimental conditions such as the type of patient tested were significantly different than in the present research.

2)   interpreting results

Regardless of the source of data, the results reported from research using historical controls tend to exaggerate the effectiveness of a new drug treatment. In a review of similar treatments tested in which both randomized control and historical control designs were used, it was concluded that the results of the trials were different based on the type of control group present. The new treatment was found effective in 84% of the trials that used historical controls, but in only 11% of the trials that used a randomized control design.[22]

Despite their limitations, historical controls are useful for rapidly obtaining initial impressions about a new drug treatment, particularly if the investigators emphasize the limitations involved in drawing conclusions or extrapolating the results.   These impressions may be the basis for the initial development of hypotheses that could be later verified by better designed clinical drug trials.

Historical controls are also useful in trials where there are significant ethical concerns regarding denial of the investigational drug to a group of patients. An example would be a clinical drug trial that evaluates zidovudine (AZT) in the treatment of patients with AIDS and advanced AIDS-related complex where the diagnosis of the condition under research is well established and the outcome is well known and harmful to the patients (i.e., death).[18]

Health care practitioners reviewing information obtained from clinical drug trials using historical controls should be skeptical about the value of the reported results to their clinical practice. Nevertheless, the results can be useful if certain criteria are met. The research should be directed toward evaluating the drug treatment for a specific disease that is similar to the one used in the historical control, specific objectives must be identified which are consistent with the current research, and clear differences must be established between the effect of the drug treatment in the present trial and the one used as the historical control.[7]

3)   an alternative to historical controls: meta-analysis

An acceptable alternative to the use of historical controls in assessing the effectiveness of investigational drugs is meta-analysis, which quantifies information from different clinical drug trials. Meta-analysis involves several steps. The published literature about a drug treatment is collected and reviewed. Only those clinical drug trials that meet a set of design criteria are selected. The data from the trials are pooled and the "effect size" calculated. The effect size is the estimation of the pooled difference between the investigational drug and the various control treatments. The pooled difference can be the average difference between experimental and control groups or a weighted difference which rewards better designed studies.   The statistical significance and the clinical importance of the differences are then evaluated.[19,20]

Meta-analysis is a useful technique because of its value in identifying previously undetected drug effects by pooling data to create a larger sample of patients. However, meta-analysis is not as useful if the clinical drug trials analyzed are poorly designed or if a significant number of trials have different outcome measures.[19,21]

10. Was patient assignment to experimental or control groups appropriate?

An important step in establishing experimental and control groups is the assignment of patients to each group. The most desirable approach is random assignment or allocation. A clinical drug trial that includes parallel control groups and random assignment of patients is called a randomized controlled trial (RCT) and is the standard by which all other designs are compared.[1,3,6,12,17,22-24]

Random assignment is a process by which all potential trial participants are equally likely to be allocated to either the experimental or control group. This type of assignment removes the potential of investigators to consciously or subconsciously influence how the patients are assigned. Randomization is more likely than other assignment procedures to produce trial groups that possess comparable characteristics. These characteristics are sometimes referred to as baseline variables or covariates and should be evenly distributed or balanced between the experimental and control groups. In addition, random assignment better ensures the appropriateness of the statistical tests used to analyze the data (see Chapter 17, Questions 16-18).[3,6,17,24]

a. Ethical concerns

The most frequent objection to random assignment is based on ethical considerations. The typical argument is that randomization will deprive about half of the patients in the trial from receiving the benefits of the investigational drug. Critics have charged that physicians and other health professionals engaged in clinical drug trials sacrifice the current interests of the patient participating in the trial in order to benefit all future similarly affected patients. Thus, random assignment would violate the personal obligation of physicians to use their best judgment and recommend the best treatment for patients no matter how tentative or inconclusive the data on which that judgment is based.[18,25-27]

The ethical conflict has been magnified with the increasing number of patients who suffer from AIDS. Patients with AIDS argue that the hopelessness of their situation should guarantee them access on a nonrandomized basis to drugs that offer some hope, even if randomized clinical trials have not been completed for those drugs. Although such patients recognize that the investigational drugs are potentially toxic and may have limited effectiveness, some claim the right to take those risks.[18]

It is unethical for physicians and other health professionals to engage knowingly in an activity that will result in inferior treatment for their patients. However, the most ethical action is not as clear when the superiority of the investigational drug is not well established. The only reliable way to make this distinction in the face of incomplete information is to test the drug treatment using a randomized controlled clinical drug trial.[26]

The ethical problems of random assignment can be largely overcome if investigators adhere to a set of well-established guidelines. The patient needs to have a free choice whether or not to take part in the clinical drug trial. This choice is often referred to as informed consent. A data-monitoring mechanism also is needed so that the trial can be discontinued if the greater efficacy or toxicity of the investigational drug treatment is clearly demonstrated. Additionally, the trial must be designed to have a definite chance of answering the question about the relative effectiveness and safety of the drug.[18,26-27]

The most important justification for random assignment of patients to experimental or control groups is the existence of a scientific and medical consensus that the investigational drug has not yet been shown to be superior to standard or existing drug treatment. This principle is difficult to apply because of the tendency of physicians and other health professionals to try newer drug treatments with the hope that their patients will benefit. Thus, random assignment should be done most often in the early phases of new drug investigations when information is generally lacking about the relative superiority of the investigational drug and it cannot be plausibly argued that patients are at serious risk of being denied a more efficacious and safe drug treatment.[18,26-27]

b. Types of randomization schemes

There are many approaches to the random assignment of patients to experimental and control groups. Some methods have a fixed or pre-specified assignment procedure while other approaches adapt the random assignment process as the clinical drug trial progresses. The most common types of the former method are simple, blocked, and stratified randomization. The most common type of the latter techniques is the biased coin method.[1,17]

   1) simple randomization

Simple randomization schemes involve a pre-arranged sequence of assignments which are random in order and in which each patient has an equal chance of being allocated to the experimental or control group. The advantage of simple randomization is that it is easy to implement. The major disadvantage is a greater possibility that the baseline characteristics of the resultant experimental and control groups may be different, particularly if the sample or group size is small. In larger trials the statistical law of large numbers reduces the chance of serious imbalance, but smaller trials are more vulnerable to potential differences in baseline characteristics (see Chapter 17, Question 20). In fact, it has been recommended by some that simple randomization schemes not be used in trials with a target sample size of under 200 patients.[1,6,17,28]

An example of an important difference occurring between the experimental and control groups after simple randomization was noted in a clinical drug trial that compared indoprofen with pentazocine in the treatment of post-traumatic pain.[29] Sixty patients suffering from pain due to fractures or serious sprains were randomly assigned to receive either the drug treatment or a placebo. Baseline measures were taken on self-assessment of pain severity (Table 15-1).

Table 15-1. Baseline Self-Assessment of Pain Severity[29]

Study Group	Pain Assessment[a]
Indoprofen	3.45
Pentazocine	3.10
Placebo	3.10

[a] Average assessment of the severity of pain was made by the patient based on a scale of 0 to 4 with 0=no pain, 1=mild pain, 2=moderate pain, 3=severe pain, 4=unbearable pain.

As indicated in Table 15-1, the mean pre-treatment pain assessment for the indoprofen group was higher despite the use of randomization. Because pain severity was the major outcome measured in this trial, the baseline differences among the groups could affect the trial results. Fortunately, the investigators were able to minimize the baseline differences using a statistical technique known as analysis of covariance (see Chapter 17, Questions 15, 18).

One easy approach to adjusting for errors in simple random assignment is to re-do the procedure and replace the old assignment with the new one. This approach is known as replacement randomization and may be impractical in clinical drug trials that involve sequential enrollment of patients.[1]

2) blocked randomization

Blocked randomization (also called permuted blocked randomization) is often used to offset imbalances in the trial groups by organizing the patients into numerical "blocks" such as four or eight individuals.[1,6,17,24] The order in which the treatments are assigned in each block is randomized and this process is repeated for consecutive blocks until all patients are assigned. For example, if the investigators want to ensure equality after every four individuals, blocks of four are created. The investigational drug assignment would be randomly arranged within each block as demonstrated in Table 15-2.

Table 15-2. Typical Assignment Sequence in a Randomized Block Design

Block (contains four patients)	Sequence[a]
One	E-C-C-E
Two	C-C-E-E
Three	E-C-E-C

[a] E represents the hypothetical random assignment to the experimental group. C represents the hypothetical random assignment to the control group.

As indicated in Table 15-2, the trial groups at the end of each block would be equal in number. Although baseline patient characteristics may be different early in the process, the groups should become more similar as the number of patients assigned increases.

Blocked randomization techniques are useful in clinical drug trials where the type or sources of patients recruited change during the entry period. This technique is also more likely to ensure balanced groups in clinical drug trials where premature termination of the trial could occur.

A potential problem with blocked randomization occurs when the investigators know the size of the blocks prior to randomization. Thus, the assignment of the last person entered in each block would be known and could distort the assignment process. Solutions to this problem include using blinding techniques, avoiding blocks of two patients, or varying the blocking factor so that it is difficult to determine where blocks start and end.

A sophisticated and commonly used blocked randomization scheme is the Latin square design in which the number of different drugs (or drug dosage schedules) equals the number of patients or blocks.[1,30] The result is referred to as an "N x N" (e.g., 4 x 4) arrangement where N is number of treatments, patients, or groups. For example, a 5 x 5 Latin square design was used in a clinical drug trial that compared the hypnotic activity of five different drug treatments: single doses of flurazepam (15 mg), loprazolam (0.5, 1, and 2 mg) and placebo.[31] The sequence of administration of the different drug treatments was randomized so that five groups of patients (12 in each group) received a single dose of one of the drugs one night per week for five weeks. Although the actual sequence of administration was not published, a possible order is described in Table 15-3.

Table 15-3.   Possible Latin Square Design for the Study of Flurazepam and Loprazolam[31]

Week	Study Group				
	1	2	3	4	5
1	$L_{0.5}$	$L_{1.0}$	$L_{2.0}$	F	P
2	$L_{1.0}$	$L_{0.5}$	P	$L_{2.0}$	F
3	$L_{2.0}$	F	$L_{0.5}$	P	$L_{1.0}$
4	F	P	$L_{1.0}$	$L_{0.5}$	$L_{2.0}$
5	P	$L_{2.0}$	F	$L_{1.0}$	$L_{0.5}$

F = Flurazepam 15 mg   P = Placebo $L_{0.5}$ = Loprazolam 0.5 mg
$L_{1.0}$ = Loprazolam 1 mg
$L_{2.0}$ = Loprazolam 2 mg

An important advantage of the Latin square design is that it can efficiently control against the influence of a number of important factors (e.g., the sequence of administration and type of drug treatment used) while using relatively small numbers of patients. The major disadvantage of this design is that it assumes that the factors do not "interact" (i.e., influence each other). The Latin square design also requires a somewhat more complex randomization scheme.[24]

3)   stratified randomization

Stratified randomization is another approach to solving problems associated with random assignment and involves classifying patients according to one or more important factors (e.g., age, gender, race, medical setting, medical condition) before assignment.   After classification, the patients are randomly assigned to the experimental or control groups. This type of randomization should be used instead of simple randomization when the clinical drug trial consists of small sample sizes in order to minimize the likelihood of producing dissimilar study groups.[1,6,8,17,24]

Stratified randomization is sometimes used to control for a factor that the investigator believes could interfere with interpretation of the reported results. This approach was illustrated in a clinical drug trial comparing benoxaprofen with ibuprofen in the treatment of osteoarthritis (knee or hip).[32] In this trial, the investigators believed that older patients may react differently to the drugs than younger patients. In addition, they also believed that the location of the arthritis (i.e., knee or hip) may affect the drug response. Thus, patients were stratified according to age (over or under 60 years) and location of the osteoarthritic joint (joint or hip). Patients within each of these four groups were randomly assigned to receive either benoxaprofen or ibuprofen. Although no significant differences appeared when the age groups were analyzed separately, the benoxaprofen effect was more pronounced in the knee joint compared with the hip.

4)   adaptive randomization (biased coin and urn method)

An alternative to using the fixed or pre-specified randomization schemes already described is a method in which the assignment process changes as the trial progresses. This process is sometimes referred to as adaptive randomization and includes the biased coin and urn methods of assignment. Biased coin assignment involves adjusting the randomization procedure so that the study group with the smallest number of patients will have a higher probability of having the next available study patient randomized to it. The major advantage of the biased coin method is that it protects against severe differences among the study group on key characteristics.[17] The urn method of randomization is a type of biased coin design that is particularly useful for studies with small sample sizes.[28]

5)   nonrandomization

While randomized assignment of patients is very desirable, many clinical drug trials will involve nonrandomized assignment techniques such as systematic or judgment assignment. The systematic method involves selecting and matching patients based on factors such as date of birth, date of appearance at the study site, or alternate numbers (i.e., odd/even). A version of the systematic approach is the assignment of pairs matched on the key factors described previously. Although systematic assignment reduces the possibility of biased allocation of patients, it can be compromised if the investigator eliminates potential patients based on advanced awareness of what drug treatment the patient is expected to receive.[1,24]

Judgment assignment is based on an assessment by the study investigator or the patient's physician as to which group the patient should be assigned. The major disadvantage of this approach is that the individual responsible for the assignment may consciously or subconsciously create significantly different experimental or control groups. Even when judgment assignment is based on "objective" assessments such as laboratory tests, it is impossible prior to the clinical drug trial to be aware of all the important factors that may make the trial groups respond differently to the drug treatment.[1,17]

Nonrandomized assignment of patients occurred in a trial comparing the effectiveness of cefaclor to that of amoxicillin in the treatment of urinary tract infections in a chronic disease hospital.[33] The result of the assignment was groups of unequal size: 25 in the experimental and 36 in the control group. In addition, a comparison of the two groups of patients indicated a significant difference in the causative organisms of urinary tract infection (Table 15-4). The presence of *Klebsiella* (which were resistant to amoxicillin) and a lower percentage of *E. coli* in the cefaclor group could have affected the response to the antibiotic and altered the comparability of the study groups.

Table 15-4. Distribution of Causative Organisms by Study Group[33]

Causative Organism	Cefaclor	Amoxicillin
E. coli	53%	79%
Klebsiella	16%	0%
Proteus	13%	17%
Enterococci	8%	4%
Miscellaneous	10%	0%

c.   Evaluation of assignment methods

Ideally, investigators should describe exactly how patients were assigned to the experimental or control groups. Terms such as "random allocation" or "random trial" are appropriate in contrast to terms such as "without conscious bias", "systematic assignment" or "allocation at the investigator's discretion."[34,35] It is also important for the health care practitioner to distinguish between the random "selection" of patients, which refers to the enrollment of trial participants, and random "assignment", which refers to the allocation of those already enrolled to the experimental and control groups.

Regardless of whether randomization is used in the patient assignment process, baseline comparisons of the study groups should be reported. Baseline comparisons should include important characteristics that may influence the trial results such as age, gender, race, medical condition, medical setting, or the presence of concurrent drug therapy.[6]

11. Were adequate blinding techniques utilized?

A primary objective when designing a clinical drug trial is to minimize the influence of patient or investigator bias on the results. This bias can be defined as the conscious or subconscious prejudices of the trial participants and/or investigators toward interpreting events in a certain manner. A specific bias that needs to be addressed in designing a clinical drug trial would be the temptation to inaccurately record improvement in signs or symptoms attributed to treatment with the investigational drug.[36,37]

Protection against patient or investigator bias is accomplished through the use of single-blinded and double-blinded designs. Usually in a single-blinded trial, the investigators, but not the patients, are aware of which treatment is being administered. A less frequent variation would be for the investigator, but not the patient, to be unaware of what drug is being given. In a double-blinded trial, neither the patient nor the investigator is aware of which treatment the patient has received until the code is broken or the results are ready to be analyzed. The typical design of clinical drug trials is double-blinded and is usually accomplished by giving the control group a "placebo" (which could be an active drug or inert substance) that is made to look, taste and smell like the investigational drug so that both the investigator and patient are masked from identifying the actual treatment.[3,37]

Although recommended for the majority of clinical drug trials, blinding techniques are most appropriate for those trials where the measurement of patient response can be interpreted subjectively. Blinding techniques are also valuable for those trials in which knowledge of the drug used may affect the way the results are interpreted or the manner in which care is administered to the patient.[3]

a. Investigator bias

Even the most well-intended investigator can inadvertently interpret the trial results in a way that will be consistent with pre-trial personal interests. The opposite effect may also occur: the investigator overcompensates for potential biases by interpreting positive drug effects in a negative way.[37] The potential for bias increases as the involvement of the investigator in the measurement process increases (e.g., assessment of pain, the severity of possible side effects, or improvement in moods).[3]

Although all aspects of the clinical drug trial should be protected against investigator bias, achieving this goal may not always be possible. Masking the drug effect would be very difficult in trials in which one or more of the drug actions is well known. This problem was illustrated in a trial of the effects of the cardiovascular drug propranolol in reducing mortality of post-myocardial infarction patients. Physicians were able to guess whether the patient was taking the drug or placebo approximately 60% of the time because of their knowledge of pharmacological effects of propranolol.[36]

b.   Patient bias

Biased patient response to an investigational drug is commonly called the placebo effect. The placebo effect usually involves patients responding to what they think the investigator wishes to hear or see. Placebo effects may mask or distort the actual effect of the investigational drug.[3,38] Almost every patient-investigator encounter in a clinical drug trial has a symbolic dimension that could produce a placebo effect. The desired success of the treatment can be felt so strongly by one or both of the parties involved that objectivity cannot be guaranteed. In addition, the act of giving a drug treatment can be a strong stimulus in itself.[37,39] Thus, it is not surprising that placebos have been shown to alter virtually any disease process that can be reversed. The placebo effect involves a wide variety of responses, ranging from "subjective" responses such as mood changes to "objective" responses such as the spontaneous disappearance of warts (Table 15-5).

Table 15-5. Biological/Disease Processes Affected by Placebo Effect[35]

Fever	Post-operative pain
Headache	Blood cell count
Cough reflex	Vasomotor function
Common cold	Adrenal gland
Insomnia	Gastric secretion/motility
Mood changes	Blood pressure
Angina	Respiratory rates
Warts	Pupil movement

Some investigators have estimated that about one-third of patients display a placebo effect in response to drug treatment. Predicting who will exhibit this behavior is difficult because of the lack of agreement on what constitutes a placebo effect.[38,39] The effect can be influenced by the nature of the drug treatment being compared. Patients are more likely to identify a placebo if the investigational drug has prominent therapeutic or toxic effects. In a trial of this phenomenon, patients were asked to guess whether they received a placebo or phenylpropanolamine, a drug used as an adjunct for weight control. While the effect of phenylpropanolamine on appetite suppression is modest, the drug has prominent side effects such as dry mouth and heart palpitations. Based on the prominence of these side effects, 75% of the patients receiving the placebo correctly guessed their treatment compared to only 43% of the patients receiving the phenylpropanolamine.[40]

When the drug side effects are not as prominent, patients have a tendency to believe they are receiving the investigational drug rather than the placebo. In a clinical drug trial of the effects of the cardiovascular drug propranolol (which has a low incidence of side effects), patients taking the drug were more likely to guess correctly (64%) than those taking the placebo (41%).[36]

c.   Assessment of blinding techniques

Investigators generally indicate when they have used blinding techniques in the clinical drug trial. The absence of any reference to these techniques in the description of the trial design should be sufficient evidence that blinding methods were not used. In addition, the health care practitioner should be wary of vague or misleading terms used by the investigators when indicating if blinding techniques were used. An example is the use of the term "open label" which generally means that both the investigator and the patient were aware of the drugs used in the trial. However, the term is not widely known and could mislead the health care practitioner unfamiliar with the expression.

It is desirable in published research papers for the trial investigator to describe the blinding techniques comprehensively. The description should include information on how the experimental and control drugs (or placebo) were made to look identical and whether they were administered in a similar fashion. It would also be helpful to describe how the results were measured and the extent of investigator involvement in those measures.[3,36]

Few investigators report the success or failure of their blinding techniques. Problems with blinding are more prominent when single blind methods are used because of the greater likelihood of an informed participant (e.g., a member of the research staff) revealing critical information about the clinical drug trial design to the patient. Blinding techniques are usually desirable in clinical drug trials for the treatment of conditions in which spontaneous variation or remission is common (e.g., rheumatoid arthritis, ulcerative colitis, angina, or peptic ulcer disease). The techniques are also more likely to be effective when indirect measures such as labratory tests or X-rays are used. These measures are less likely to reveal the identity of the drug treatment.[3,37,40]

References

1.   Pocock SJ. Clinical trials: a practical approach. New York: Wiley & Sons, 1983:4,50-90.
2.   Polk RE, Hepler CD. Controversies in antimicrobial therapy: critical analysis of clinical trials. *Am J Hosp Pharm* 1986;43:630-40.
3.   Cuddy PG, Elenbaas RM, Elenbaas JK. Evaluating the medical literature. Part I: abstract, introduction, methods. *Ann Emerg Med* 1983;12:549-55.
4.   Guyatt G, Sackett D, Taylor DW, Chong J, Roberts R, Pubsley S. Determining optimal therapy-randomized trials in individual patients. *N Engl J Med* 1986;314:889-92.
5.   Campbell MJ, Machin D. Medical statistics: a common sense approach. New York: John Wiley & Sons, 1990:5-13.
6.   Lavori PW, Louis TA, Bailar JC, Polansky M. Designs for experiments-parallel comparisons of treatment. *N Engl J Med* 1983;309:1291-8.
7.   Bailar JC, Louis TA, Lavori PW, Polansky M. Statistics in practice: studies without internal controls. *N Engl J Med* 1984;311:156-62.

8. Lachin JM. Statistical properties of randomization in clinical trials. *Controlled Clinical Trials* 1988;9:289-311.

9. Yusuf S, Held P, Teo KK. Selection of patients for randomized controlled trials: implications of wide or narrow eligibility criteria. *Stat Med* 1990;9:73-86.

10. MaKuch R, Johnson M. Issues in planning and interpreting active control equivalence studies. *J Clin Epidemiol* 1989;42:503-11.

11. Ritter JM. Placebo-controlled, double-blind clinical trials can impede medical progress. *Lancet* 1980;1:1126-7.

12. Kitler ME. The changing face of clinical trials. *J Hypertension* 1988;6(suppl 1):S73-S80.

13. Gehlbach SH. Interpreting the medical literature: a clinician's guide. New York, Macmillan Publishing Company, 1988:70-74.

14. Louis TA, Lavori PW, Bailar JC, Polansky M. Crossover and self-controlled designs in clinical research. *N Engl J Med* 1984;310:24-31.

15. Berezuk GP, Schondelmeyer SW, Seidenfeld JJ, Jones WN, Bootman JL. Clinical comparison of albuterol, isoetharine, and metaproterenol given by aerosol inhalation. *Clin Pharm* 1983;2:129-34.

16. United States Pharmacopeia. Drug information for the health professional. 13th edition. Rockville. United States Pharmacopeial Convention, Inc., 1993.

17. Friedman LM, Furberg CD, DeMets DL. Fundamentals of clinical trials. 2nd ed. Littleton, MA:PSG Publishing, 1985:34-65.

18. Veatch RM. Drug research in humans: the ethics of nonrandomized access. *Clin Pharm* 1989;8:366-70.

19. Einarson TR, McGhan WF, Bootman JL, Sabers DL. Meta-analysis: quantitative integration of independent research results. *Am J Hosp Pharm* 1985;42:1957-64.

20. Boissel JP, Blanchard J, Panak E, Peyrieux JC, Sacks H. Considerations for the meta-analysis of randomized clinical trials. *Controlled Clinical Trials* 1989;10:254-81.

21. Sacks HS, Berrier J, Reitman D, Ancona-Berk VA, Chalmers TC. Meta-analysis of randomized controlled trials. *N Engl J Med* 1987;316:450-5.

22. Sacks H, Chalmers TC, Smith H. Sensitivity and specificity of clinical trials: randomized versus historical controls. *Arch Intern Med* 1983;143:753-5.

23. Inglefinger FJ. The randomized clinical trial. *N Engl J Med* 1972;287:100-1.

24. Hallstrom A, Davis K. Imbalance in treatment assignments in stratified blocked randomization. *Controlled Clinical Trials* 1988;9:375-82.

25. Hellman S, Hellman DS. Of mice but not men: problems of the randomized clinical trial. *N Engl J Med* 1991;324:1585-9.

26. Passamani E. Clinical trials-are they ethical? *N Engl J Med* 1991;324:1589-92.

27. Kodish E. Ethical considerations in randomized controlled clinical trials. *Cancer* 1990;65:2400-4.

28. Wei LJ, Lachin JM. Properties of the urn randomization in clinical trials. *Controlled Clinical Trials* 1988;9:345-64.

29. Soave G, Lavezzari M, Ferrati G, Sacchetti G. Indoprofen and pentazocine in post-traumatic pain. A double-blind, parallel-group comparative trial. *J Int Med Res* 1983;11:354-57.

30. Neter J, Wasserman W, Kutner MH. Applied linear statistical models. Boston: RD Irwin 1990: 1083-8.

31. Elie R, Caille G, Levasseur FA, Gareau J. Comparative hypnotic activity of single doses of loprazolam, flurazepam, and placebo. *J Clin Pharmacol* 1983;23:32-6.
32. Tyson VCH, Gynne A. A comparative trial of benoxaprofen and ibuprofen in osteoarthritis in general practice. *J Rheumatology* 1980;7(suppl 6):132-8.
33. Lindon R. Comparison of cefaclor and amoxicillin in the treatment of urinary infections in a chronic disease hospital. *Postgraduate Med* 1979;55(suppl 4):67-9.
34. Sackett DL. How to read clinical journals: I. Why to read them and how to start reading them critically. *CMA Journal* 1981;124:555-8.
35. Mosteller F, Gilbert JP, McPeek B. Reporting standards and research strategies for controlled trials. *Controlled Clinical Trials* 1980;1:37-58.
36. Byington RP, Curb JD, Mattson ME. Assessment of double-blindness at the conclusion of the beta blocker heart attack trial. *JAMA* 1985;253:1733-6.
37. Ederer F. Patient bias, investigator bias, and the double-masked procedure in clinical trials. *Am J Med* 1975;58:295-9.
38. Bush PJ. The placebo effect. *J Am Pharm Assoc* 1974;NS14:671-4.
39. Brody H. The placebo response (Parts I-II). *Drug Ther* 1986(July):106,115-122,131.
40. Moscucci M, Byrne L, Weintraub M, Cox C. Blinding, unblinding, and the placebo effect: an analysis of patients' guesses of treatment assignment in a double-blind clinical trial. *Clin Pharmacol Ther* 1987;41:259-65.

Checklist Questions

12. What methods were used to ensure the quality of the measures used in the clinical drug trial?

13. How appropriate were the measures of drug effects?

Discussion

Gathering data regarding the effects of the investigational drug in a clinical trial involves the selection of a set of measures that properly evaluate the drug's efficacy and safety for the disease under research. While standard sets of measures sometimes exist, more often investigators develop their own or modify existing ones. Thus, the information acquired by the investigator may be faulty and not entirely representative of the true patient outcomes induced by the investigational drug. Two common problems that occur in the measurement process are the use of poor quality measures or those that are not appropriate for assessing the investigational drug's efficacy or safety.

Explanation of Checklist Questions

12. What methods were used to ensure the quality of the measures used in the trial?

Most measures used in clinical drug trials are approximations of the drug's effect because the specific outcomes often cannot be measured directly. The indirect approach makes the measurement process prone to two types of measurement errors: those that occur in an unpredictable manner (i.e., random measurement error) and those that occur in a biased, predictable fashion (i.e., systematic measurement error). An example of a random measurement error would be the subjective evaluation of lung X-rays in order to assess the effectiveness of anti-tubercular drugs. The evaluation may be unpredictable because of a lack of consensus about what type of radiologic evidence represents a "cure" for tuberculosis. In contrast, systematic measurement errors are illustrated by the use of observers who anticipate a patient's response to drug treatment. Investigators with preconceived notions about an investigational drug's effectiveness are more likely to be influenced by those impressions when interpreting the results. Both types of measurement errors can influence the evaluation of an investigational drug's efficacy and safety but systematic measurement errors are usually more damaging unless properly controlled.[1-3]

a.   Reducing measurement error

Both random and systematic measurement error are reduced by ensuring that the most reliable and valid measures are used in assessing drug effects (Table 16-1).

Table 16-1. Description of Reliability and Validity of Measures

Characteristic	Description
Reliability (reproducibility)	Ability of measure to produce the same result if used more than once.
Validity	The extent to which a measure assesses what is supposed to be measured.

The evaluation of the reliability or reproducibility of a measure should focus on the agreement among a set of repeated measures on the same patient. Two measures of a patient's blood pressure taken a month apart should be roughly the same if the patient's status has not changed. The reliability of a measure is often confused with the measure's accuracy. However, the two concepts are not interchangeable. Accuracy is a general term that refers to the exactness or the precision of the measure, while reliability applies to its consistency or stability.[3-5]

The examination of a measure's validity focuses on what is being considered and whether the test is actually measuring the right concept.[6-8] For example, the assessment of the clinical effectiveness of an antibiotic is sometimes based on the pharmacokinetics of the drug, its *in vitro* effects, or its pharmacologic activity. While these measures are important characteristics, they do not replace the more valid measures of clinical effectiveness: eradication of the harmful bacteria or reduction of associated symptoms.[9] A test or measure that is not reliable cannot be valid. However, invalid measures can be reliable.[6]

A variety of approaches are used to improve the reliability and validity of the measurement process and reduce the likelihood of measurement error (Table 16-2). The use of these approaches to measure the investigational drug's efficacy and safety should be explained comprehensively and clearly in any description of a clinical drug trial.

Table 16-2. Common Procedures Used to Reduce the Likelihood of Measurement Error

Procedure	Effect on Measurement Process
Standardized measures	Consistent interpretation
Sensitive measures	Increased detection of change
Blind observers and patients	Reduction in observer bias
Multiple measures	Improved reliability and validity

b.   Standardized measures

Clinical drug trials for the treatment of a particular medical condition often vary in the types of measures used, making comparison of the results difficult. Assessment of an anti-arthritic drug's effectiveness could vary, depending on how the response of the inflamed joint (i.e., joint count) is measured. The drug may be more effective in a trial which measured the number of "tender" joints compared to a trial that counted the number of "swollen" joints.[10]

Even when the measures are similar, few investigators describe the exact manner in which the measures are used.[2,7] An example of a clear description occurred in a trial comparing the effectiveness of norfloxacin with co-trimoxazole in the treatment of urinary tract infections.[11] Therapeutic effectiveness of the two antibiotics was represented by measures of the number of bacteria eradicated in the urine (i.e., bacterial cure) and relief of symptoms associated with urinary tract infections (i.e., clinical cure). The bacterial cure was measured by a standardized urinalysis in which the urine collection scheme was specified clearly by the investigators (i.e., two mid-stream urine specimens). The clinical cure was assessed by blinded observations and physical examination. Both measures were performed four times during the trial and at the appropriate time interval for allowing the investigational drug to reach its optimal activity level.

c.   Sensitive measures

The sensitivity of a measure refers to its ability to accurately assess the magnitude of change that occurred. Clinical drug trials often fail to show a particular result because the measurements used are not sufficiently sensitive to detect the changes in the desired outcome. In the treatment of arthritis, trials that use radiographic findings to assess joint healing often failed to reveal success compared with more sensitive measures such as counting the number of improved joints.[10]

However, extremely sensitive measures may also cause problems. Such measures are likely to detect small differences between the experimental and control group which could be clinically unimportant. The overly optimistic investigator may choose to interpret and report these differences as clinically important when, in fact, they are not.[12]

d.   Blind observers and patients

Two major sources of systematic measurement error in clinical drug trials are the bias of the investigator in interpreting events and the bias of the patient in reporting results. Thus, keeping the observers and the patients blind to the type of drug treatment used is an effective way to reduce these influences (see Chapter 15, Question 11). If the type of drug treatment under investigation prevents blinding of the investigator, observers independent from the research team should be used to measure trial outcomes.[2,13-14]

e.   Multiple measures

Utilizing multiple measures will often reduce the likelihood of measurement error by improving the reliability and validity of the measurement process. Multiple measures are used in clinical drug trials in order to assess all important aspects of the patient's response and to avoid missing any evidence of benefit.[7,10]

The use of multiple measures is illustrated in a trial that compared the effectiveness of piroxicam versus naproxen in the treatment of rheumatoid arthritis (Table 16-3).[15]

Table 16-3. Measures Used to Assess the Therapeutic Effect of the Anti-Arthritic Drugs Piroxicam and Naproxen[15]

Patient Self-assessment[a]	Night-time activity General physical limitation Specific daily activity Duration of morning stiffness
Investigator Assessment[a]	Number of swollen joints Number of painful joints at rest and at motion American Rheumatism Association functional class Grip strength Detailed assessment of total joint pain
Overall Therapeutic Effect[a]	By patient By investigator

[a]   Both the patients and the investigators were blinded to the identity of the drug treatment.

As indicated in Table 16-3, 11 different measures were used to assess the therapeutic effect of the two anti-arthritic drugs. In addition, the results were obtained from two sources: the patient and the investigator.

Unfortunately, the use of multiple measures can be detrimental if the strategy relies more on the number of measures used than on the quality of each measure. Use of a large number of poor measures may result in different findings, which could make assessment of the drug effect difficult. The choice of which measures to believe can be confusing, especially if they differ in quality. A better solution would be to carefully choose measures that are most relevant, sensitive to change, and not duplicative of other measures used in the trial.[10]

13. How appropriate were the measures of drug effects?

In a clinical drug trial, the assessment of drug effects involves focusing on the advantages and disadvantages of using the drug in a selected patient population. The advantages are the expected therapeutic effects, while the disadvantages include possible adverse drug reactions, drug sensitivities, or drug use problems such as noncompliance.[1,3,16,17] The appropriateness of the measures used for each of these effects can greatly influence how the trial results are interpreted.

a. Measures of therapeutic effects

Measures of therapeutic effects usually are derived from the goals of the drug treatment and the disease under investigation. In general, the goals are the cure of the disease, relief of symptoms, the prevention of disease progression, or the reduction of patient mortality.[18] While these goals are clear, selection of the appropriate measures may be difficult due to reasons such as unavailability, expense, potential harm to the patient, or the complexity of the measure.

The difficulty in selecting appropriate measures is illustrated by the evaluation of the therapeutic effect of drug treatment for Irritable Bowel Syndrome (IBS). Because IBS is associated with a wide variety of symptoms of the gastrointestinal tract, investigators often measure drug effectiveness by using an extensive battery of specific tests (15 or greater) of poor individual quality or an overall measure which combines numerous single measures. Neither of these approaches is desirable. The ideal set of measures would assess improvement in the important clinical features of the disease (e.g., relief of abdominal cramping or less frequent watery bowel movements) and in patient attitudes or feelings. The best evidence of efficacy would be significant improvement in measures of patient feelings and most of the efficacy measures, especially if the pattern made clinical sense. If significant improvements were found in only a small number of the specific measures, then conclusions regarding the investigational drug's effectiveness would be tentative at best.[18]

Another set of measures sometimes used to evaluate drug efficacy assesses the impact of the drug on the other aspects of the patient's lifestyle. These tests are often referred to as "quality of life" measures and are especially useful for diseases that are asymptomatic (e.g., hypertension) or not immediately life-threatening (e.g., arthritis).[19] In addition, quality of life measures represent another source of information about the efficacy and safety of the investigational drug. This set of measures generally consists of two major components: daily functioning and patient perceptions (Table 16-4).[20]

Table 16-4. Dimensions of Quality of Life[13]

Daily Functioning	Social interactions with friends, family, etc.
	Physical mobility
	Emotional stability or self-control
	Intellectual capability
Patient Perceptions	Life satisfaction or perceived well-being
	Health status (absolute or relative)

As indicated in Table 16-4, the functional component refers to the ability of the patient to perform certain acts within their environment. The measures of daily functioning tend to be based on patient self-reporting and objective or subjective investigator observations. The perceptual component of quality of life concentrates on the patients' attitudes toward their health and life. Measures of the perceptual component of quality of life tend to be more subjective than the functional component. Both types of quality of life measures tend to be broad instead of disease-specific. Thus, they are sometimes difficult to relate to the clinical measures of drug efficacy and safety performed at the same time.

b.   Measures of adverse drug reactions

The measurement of adverse drug reactions (ADRs) is a crucial but complex step in the evaluation of drug treatment.   Measuring ADRs is difficult because of a lack of understanding regarding why they occur.   Unlike the few and generally well-defined outcome measures for therapeutic effects, there could be many possible ADRs that need to be monitored in a clinical drug trial. In addition, the assessment of ADRs is often viewed as of secondary importance to the investigators and less attention is devoted to effectively measuring ADRs when developing the trial design.[19-23] ADRs are typically measured by the methods shown in Table 16-5.[19-20] The most common measures of ADRs are observer or self-reported patient complaints that may be associated with the drug treatment.

Table 16-5. Common Measures of ADRs Used in Clinical Drug Trials[19,20]

- Self-reported patient complaints
- Observer-reported patient complaints
- Laboratory measurements and X-rays
- Subjects who withdraw from trials because of possible ADRs
- Subjects who require drug dosage reductions

The major limitation of all ADR measures is the lack of consensus regarding how to best interpret the information collected.   Attempts have been made to standardize the measures by identifying general criteria that should be used during the process (Table 16-6). However, there is still a lack of consensus about how the criteria should be used in identifying specific ADRs.[22,24]

Table 16-6. General Criteria Used for Identifying ADRs[22]

- Onset of the ADR compared to administration of the drug
- Course of the ADR after discontinuation of the drug
- Course of the ADR without discontinuation of the drug
- Patient response when the drug is re-administered
- Presence of clinical signs, symptoms characteristic of the ADR
- Presence of patient risk factors that could precipitate the ADR
- Presence of concurrent drugs that could precipitate the ADR
- Possible nondrug factors that could precipitate the ADR
- Specific tests for the ADR are used

One possible approach to improving the identification of specific ADRs is the use of "consensus conferences." Consensus conferences involve participants responsible for evaluating drug safety such as regulatory officials, health care practitioners, and drug manufacturers meeting to establish precise criteria for identifying ADRs. Examples of the types of criteria developed by a consensus conference are listed in Table 16-7.

Table 16-7. Consensus Conference Criteria for Drug-Induced Reduction of White Blood Cells (Agranulocytosis)[22]

- White blood cell (WBC) count was normal before the drug was administered
- WBC count returns to normal after the drug was discontinued
- Other blood factors (e.g., red blood cells, platelets) are normal during administration of the drug

---

In addition to defining the criteria used to assess an ADR, the appropriate length of the observation period should be established. ADRs occur relatively infrequently and are more likely to be identified as the length of the clinical drug trial increases.[20] The duration of the observation period is particularly important for drugs that are expected to be administered for extended time periods. Examples of such drugs are those that are used to treat hypertension or congestive heart failure.[25]

c. Measures of patient compliance

Patient compliance is an important part of clinical drug trials, particularly those involving ambulatory patients. The failure of patients to take their medications correctly during the trial can dramatically influence the interpretation of the results. For example, the therapeutic efficacy of an investigational drug may be overestimated because the investigator failed to account for patients who dropped out due to noncompliance with the drug regimen. In addition, the toxicity of the drug may be underestimated if the patients intentionally reduced the amount of medication they ingested during the drug trial. Thus, the extrapolation of trial results could be limited if the potential noncompliance with the drug in the clinical setting is not evaluated accurately.[26-27]

The investigator should discuss the methods used in the trial to offset the possible negative influence of patient noncompliance. Some traditional methods include the use of pill counts, monitoring serum drug levels, urine analysis of drug metabolites, use of drug "markers," patient self-reporting and physician estimations of noncompliance. Because these methods are limited in their ability to estimate compliance or are difficult to implement, other more accurate measures such as the use of electronic measuring devices are now being used in many clinical drug trials.[28-30]

d. Description of measures

Publications describing clinical drug trials should include a clear and comprehensive explanation of the measures used to evaluate the effects of the drug treatment.[31] Most clinical drug trials use a comprehensive set of measures to assess therapeutic effect. However, the measurement of ADRs and patient compliance are often not as comprehensive. A typical measurement plan was demonstrated in a clinical drug trial that compared the effectiveness of amoxicillin with that of cefaclor in the treatment of urinary tract infections (Table 16-8).[32]

Table 16-8. Measures Used to Assess Drug Efficacy and Safety in the Treatment of Urinary
           Tract Infections[32]

Measure	Description and Frequency
Therapeutic Effect	
Urine cultures:	Performed at four different time intervals
Relief of symptoms:	Patient self-report at the end of treatment
Antibiotic susceptibility:	Cultured bacteria isolates at the beginning of trial
Adverse Drug Reactions	
Laboratory tests:	Before and after the trial
Patient interview:	At the end of the trial
Patient Compliance	
Pill counts:	At the end of the trial
Patient interview:	At the end of the trial

As indicated in Table 16-8, the measures of therapeutic effect appear to be emphasized more than the measures of adverse drug reactions or patient compliance. The use of urine cultures to assess eradication of bacteria is a widely accepted standard and was performed more often than any other measure. However, although laboratory tests are an acceptable measure of adverse drug reactions, they were done only twice. In addition, patient interviews for the reporting of side effects were performed only at the end of the trial and were prone to patient recall problems. A more effective method would be standardized and more frequent observations by a health care practitioner. The least comprehensive coverage was the measures of compliance. Both compliance measures were performed only at the end of the trial and are not recognized as being accurate assessments of compliance behavior.[19,20,26,30-31]

References

1. Cuddy PG, Elenbaas RM, Elenbaas JK. Evaluating the medical literature. Part I: abstract, introduction, methods. *Ann Emerg Med* 1983;12:549-55.
2. Gehlbach SH. Interpreting the medical literature: a clinician's guide. New York, Macmillan Publishing Company, 1988:83-95.
3. McAuley WJ. Applied research in gerontology. New York: Van Nostrand-Reinhold, 1987:77-103.
4. Isaacs S, Michael WB. Handbook in research and evaluation. San Diego: Edits Publishers, 1976:125.

5. Speedie SM. Reliability: the accuracy of a test. *Am J Pharm Ed* 1985;49:76-9.
6. Kimberlin CL. Characteristics desired in tests: validity. *Am J Pharm Ed* 1985;49:73-85.
7. Haynes RB. How to read clinical journals. II. To learn about a diagnostic test. *CMA Journal* 1981;124:703-10.
8. Verbrugge LM. Scientific and professional allies in validity studies. In Fowler FJ, ed. Health Survey Research Methods. Conference Proceedings Series. DHHS Publ. No. (PHS) 89:3447.
9. Polk RE, Hepler CD. Controversies in antimicrobial therapy: critical analysis of clinical trials. *Am J Hosp Pharm* 1986;43:630-40.
10. Felson DT, Anderson JJ, Meenan RF. Time for changes in design, analysis, and reporting of rheumatoid arthritis clinical trials. *Arth Rheum* 1990;33:140-9.
11. Wong WT, Chan MK, Li MK, Wong WS, Yin PD, Cheng IKP. Treatment of Urinary tract infections in Hong Kong: a comparative study of norfloxacin and co-trimoxazole. *Scan J Inf Dis* 1988;56(suppl):22-7.
12. Horwitz RI. Complexity and contradiction in clinical trial research. *Am J Med* 1987;82:498-510.
13. Franks P. Clinical trials. *Fam Med* 1988;20:443-8.
14. Riegelman RK, Hirsch RP. Studying a study and testing a test. 2nd ed. Boston: Little Brown, 1989:19-24.
15. Fenton SF, Ryan JP, Bensen WG. A double-blind, crossover, multicenter study of piroxicam and naproxen in rheumatoid arthritis. *Curr Ther Res* 1988;44:1058-70.
16. Pocock SJ. Clinical trials: a practical approach. New York: Wiley & Sons, 1983:188-91.
17. Weintraub M. How to critically assess clinical drug trials. *Drug Ther* 1982;(July):131-48.
18. Klein KB. Controlled treatment trials in the irritable bowel syndrome: a critique. *Gastroenterology* 1988;95:232-41.
19. Dimenas E, Dahlof C, Olofsson B, Wiklund I. An instrument for quantifying subjective symptoms among untreated and treated hypertensives: development and documentation. *J Clin Res Pharmacoepidem* 1990;4:205-17.
20. Friedman LM, Furberg CD, DeMets DL. Fundamentals of clinical trials. 2nd ed. Littleton, MA:PSG Publishing, 1985:147-66.
21. Brennan TA, Localio RJ, Laird NL. Reliability and validity of judgments concerning adverse events suffered by hospitalized patients. *Med Care* 1989;27:1148-58.
22. Benichou C, Danan G. Experts' opinion in causality assessment: results of consensus meetings. *Drug Info J* 1991;25:251-5.
23. Lydeck E, Blumenthal SJ, Guess HA. Twenty years of renal adverse experience reporting with Indocin®. *J Clin Res Pharmacoepidem* 1990;4:183-9.
24. Hutchinson TA, Lane DA. Assessing methods for causality assessment of suspected adverse drug reactions. *J Clin Epidem* 1989;42:5-16.
25. Kitler ME. The changing face of clinical trials. *J Hypertension* 1988;6 (suppl 1):S73-S80.
26. Kramer MS, Shapiro SH. Scientific challenges in the application of randomized trials. *JAMA* 1984;252:2739-45.
27. Freedman LS. The effect of partial noncompliance on the power of a clinical trial. *Controlled Clinical Trials* 1990;11:157-68.
28. Meichenbaum D, Turk DC. Facilitating treatment adherence: a practitioner's guidebook. New York, New York: Plenum Press 1987:31-40.
29. Roth HP. Measurement of compliance. *Pat Educ Coun* 1987;10:107-16.

30. Averbuch M, Weintraub M, Pollock DJ. Compliance assessment in clinical trials. *J Clin Res Pharmacoepidem* 1990;4:199-204.
31. Tugwell PX. How to read clinical journals. III. To learn the clinical course and prognosis of disease. *CMA Journal* 1981;124:869-872.
32. Jaffe AC, O'Brien CA, Reed MD, Blumer JL. Randomized comparative evaluation of Augmentin® and cefaclor in pediatric skin and soft-tissue infections. *Curr Ther Res* 1985;38:160-8.

Checklist Questions

14. *Were all protocol deviations reported and managed appropriately?*

15. *Were all patient retention and data collection problems reported and controlled in the analysis?*

16. *Were descriptive statistics used properly to describe the trial results?*

17. *Were figures, graphs, or tables used adequately to present the trial results?*

18. *Was the approach described by the investigators appropriate for analyzing possible differences between the experimental and control groups?*

19. *Were the results of the significance testing interpreted correctly?*

20. *What influence does the number of patients analyzed have on the interpretation of the reported results?*

Discussion

The results section of an original research article describes how the clinical drug trial design was implemented and what actually occurred in the trial. Much of the description in the results section is quantitative, with an emphasis on the presentation of numbers and statistics that are used to reveal relevant information about the reported results.

The central feature of a well-written results section is the effective communication of the relevant clinical findings that may be applied to clinical practice. Because it is the investigator's responsibility to ensure that the reported results are communicated clearly and concisely, the discussion should be simple in structure so that the health care practitioner can easily understand the strategy employed in the analysis and presentation of the trial data. The presentation of results should be consistent with the objectives of the clinical drug trial including a proper coverage of the measures of efficacy, safety, and compliance. Any factor which may impact the interpretation of the results, such as protocol deviations or poor retention of patients in the trial, should also be reported.[1-5]

Explanation of Checklist Questions

14. Were all protocol deviations reported and managed appropriately?

Regardless of the quality of the trial design, its implementation is likely to involve some variation from expectations. Departures from the intended design, often referred to as protocol deviations or violations, can significantly affect the quality of the data collected. Protocol deviations can be classified into those of major or minor importance. Major protocol deviations may greatly affect the results of the trial while minor protocol deviations have relatively little effect on the quality of the data collected (Table 17-1). A high incidence of protocol deviations may be an indication that the trial is poorly administered with poor cooperation from patients and investigators. Major and minor protocol deviations should be reported, particularly if they are likely to bias the interpretation of the trial results.[1,7]

Table 17-1. Examples of Major and Minor Protocol Deviations

Major	Treating patients with the wrong diagnosis
	Patient noncompliance with drug therapy
	Use of concurrent, potentially interacting medications
	Investigator or patient awareness of drug treatment protocol
Minor	Variations in the data collection procedures
	Patient noncompliance with nondrug factors such as diet or sleep

a.   Treating patients with the wrong diagnosis

The treatment of patients with the wrong diagnosis often results from poor initial assessment of the patient, failure to use the proper diagnostic tests prior to enrollment, or the use of vague selection criteria. Although clear and precise selection criteria should prevent large numbers of ineligible patients from entering the trial, a small number of such patients are often included by mistake. Ineligible patients can significantly affect the trial results in a variety of ways, especially if the number of ineligible patients is relatively large. One possible effect would be a sample of patients significantly different than the patients originally targeted by the investigators. A less likely impact could be an alteration of the comparability of the experimental and control groups through assignment of significantly more ineligible patients to one of the groups. The use of random assignment should reduce the likelihood of different groups. However, the potential for assigning more ineligible patients to one of the groups increases as the sample size decreases.[1,7]

b.   Patient noncompliance

Patient noncompliance with medication administration guidelines is a major problem in clinical drug trials involving ambulatory patients.   Noncompliance may be due to a misunderstanding of the treatment instructions, mistakes in administration of the investigational drugs, or a deliberate attempt by the patient to take the medication improperly.   Noncompliance due to patient misunderstanding is usually the result of poor communication between the investigators and the patient.   Administration errors of the drugs used in the trial may be due to the mislabeling of the drugs for a specific patient or to the dispensing of the wrong medication during a clinic visit.   Deliberate noncompliance may be caused by the presence of undesirable side effects, failed therapeutic effect, or ineffective monitoring of the patient's medication use. Discovering that a substantial number of patients do not comply with the trial guidelines for taking medications may indicate that the trial protocol is difficult for the patients to follow.   In addition, reduced patient compliance in one treatment group relative to another could result in investigators making incorrect conclusions regarding the observed differences between the investigational drugs.   The investigators may incorrectly favor one investigational drug over another or conclude that no difference exists when one actually does.[1,7-9]

c.   Use of concurrent medications

The use of concurrent medications is common in studies with ambulatory patients, especially under conditions in which the patients are likely to suffer from other medical problems. Concurrent medications are often permitted because of the ethical need to ensure that the trial patients receive proper care for all medical conditions as well as the one being investigated in the trial.   Although their use may be unrelated to the investigational drug, concurrent medications are sometimes used as part of the standard of care for the medical condition being studied, to compensate for the poor efficacy of the investigational drug, or to treat the side effects that are caused by the drug.   Examples would be the use of an adjunct pain reliever such as acetaminophen in a trial assessing the safety and efficacy of an anti-arthritic drug or the use of naloxone to reverse respiratory depression caused by narcotic drugs in a trial investigating the treatment of acute pain. All concurrent medications used in the trial should be reported because they may mask the true effects of the investigational drug.[1,7,10]

d.   Investigator awareness of the drug treatment protocol

Investigator or patient awareness of which drug treatment a particular patient is receiving would be a violation of the trial protocol in double-blinded clinical drug trials.   Although the problem may occur when the confidential code identifying the trial drugs is inappropriately opened or when the patient assignment scheme is improperly revealed, protocol deviations are also likely to occur when the investigational or control drugs have prominent therapeutic effects or adverse drug reactions. Investigator or patient awareness of the drug treatment procedures can significantly bias the collection and interpretation of the data collected and represents a serious protocol deviation (see Chapter 15, Question 11).[1,11-14]

e.   Variations in the data collection procedures

Data collection problems such as patients missing scheduled appointments or investigators failing to record patient responses at consistent times often occur during the clinical drug trial. Although such violations usually do not affect the overall interpretation of the reported results, they can be important in clinical trials of certain types of drugs. An example would be assessment of the comparative effectiveness of two inhalant bronchodilators such as albuterol and epinephrine. The duration of action of albuterol is 3 to 6 hours and that of epinephrine is 1 to 3 hours. One-hour variations in the time when data are collected could result in cases when the effects of the drugs are no longer present. Because the duration of epinephrine's effect is shorter, variations in data collection may produce results which inaccurately favor albuterol.[1,7,15]

f.   Patient noncompliance with nondrug factors

Nondrug factors that are important in clinical drug trials include the type of diet to be used and the amount of sleep time required. Patient noncompliance with these factors generally does not affect the overall interpretation of the reported results. However, noncompliance with nondrug factors may be an indirect indication of noncompliance with the drug regimen or communication problems between the trial patients and the investigators.[1,7]

15. *Were all patient retention and data collection problems reported and controlled in the analysis?*

Retaining patients is a difficult task in most clinical drug trials. Even more difficult is the collection of a complete set of data on all patients. The problems associated with patient retention and data collection are summarized in Table 17-2.

Table 17-2. Problems Associated with Patient Retention and Data Collection

Problem	Description
Ineligible patients	Patients included in the trial who were later found to not fit the selection criteria
Missing data	Incomplete collection of data for each patient in the trial
Insufficient sample size	Insufficient number of patients to properly analyze the reported results
Incomparable groups	Baseline differences between the experimental and control groups

a.   Ineligible patients

There are no clear rules regarding the handling of ineligible patients in the analysis of the reported results. Although most investigators tend to omit discussion of patients not included in the analysis, the results, along with the reasons for ineligibility, should be reported. Providing details about ineligible patients can reveal important information regarding the efficacy and safety of the investigational drug. The details are of special importance if the patients were declared ineligible because of an adverse drug reaction. Reporting the number of ineligible patients also provides information about the full range of patients considered for the clinical drug trial. Such data may be useful when applying the trial results to patients who would be using the drug in clinical practice (see Chapter 14, Question 6).[7,14]

b.   Missing data

It is inevitable in most clinical drug trials that complete data will not be collected for every patient enrolled. The frequency with which data are missing should be presented precisely and clearly in order to provide information about the quality of the trial. In addition, the potential impact of the missing data on the reported results should be assessed. In particular, inconsistencies between the number of patients reported in figures, graphs, tables, or text should be explained. Numbers that are reduced because of incomplete patient data should be clearly reconciled with the number of patients originally enrolled in the trial, especially if the reduced numbers appear in tables, figures, or graphs.[4,5,14,16]

While limited amounts of missing data from incomplete observations of patients can generally be managed, a more serious problem is the lack of data due to patient withdrawal or dropout. Patients who withdraw from a clinical drug trial are often omitted from the figures, graphs, or tables used to illustrate the reported results and are sometimes not included in the data used to evaluate the efficacy and safety of the investigational drug. The omission of these type of data can create a misleading impression about the investigational drug's efficacy and safety because the focus would be on the patients who tolerated the drug and not on the complete range of patients in the original target population. Thus, it would be unwise to draw conclusions regarding the value of an investigational drug from the reported results of a trial in which a significant number of patients have withdrawn. Even if omitting data from withdrawn patients will not affect the trial results, the investigators' failure to clearly address the withdrawal problem creates a feeling of uncertainty about the potential bias present in the interpretation of the trial findings.[14,17,18]

c.   Insufficient sample size

Investigators often fail to enroll the optimal sample size or number of patients for a clinical drug trial because of the inherent problems associated with patient enrollment. Although rarely done, the intended sample size for the trial should be described in the methods section along with the reasons why the goal was not achieved, in order to provide indirect insight into possible biases that occurred in the recruitment of patients for the trial. An example would be reporting that the enrollment goal was not met due to lack of patient interest in the trial. The lack of interest may reflect the patients' belief that the investigational drug was of insufficient value to induce them to enroll in the trial.[7,14,17]

A major reason for not meeting original patient enrollment goals is the ending of a clinical drug trial earlier than originally planned. The early completion of a trial may be due to the investigators' belief that the efficacy or safety of the investigational drug was clearly established and further testing was unnecessary. Trials may also be completed early because the enrollment period closes before the full extent of the patient dropout rate is known. Early completion of a clinical drug trial is sometimes anticipated prior to the trial and should be based on systematically planned interim assessments of the investigational drug's efficacy and safety. Because there are no established guidelines regarding when a clinical drug trial should be concluded, the potential exists for ending at the wrong time. Ending prematurely tends to exaggerate the reported results because of the tendency to stop a trial at the point when the expected differences between the investigational and control drug are greatest. It is possible that the size of the difference is a random occurrence and will probably decrease if the trial continues. Thus, any decision to halt a trial early should be dependent on pre-trial estimates of expected size or the clinical importance of the observed difference between the experimental and control groups. Once the trial begins, formalized evaluation of the efficacy and safety of the drug should be done at planned intervals by independent observers. In addition, the decision to stop early ought to be explicitly noted in the reports of the results.[19,20]

d.   Incomparable groups

The loss of patients during a clinical drug trial can affect the comparability of the patients in the experimental and control groups, resulting in a misleading interpretation of the efficacy and safety of the investigational drug. Random assignment of patients to the experimental and control groups is the most effective strategy to ensure that the groups are comparable, especially if the patients are stratified first by known influential factors such as age, gender, or race. Differences between the experimental and control groups are likely to occur in clinical drug trials with random assignment of a small number of patients, using flawed randomization procedures, or with nonrandomized assignment (see Chapter 15, Question 10).[1,14,21,22]

Regardless of the assignment method, investigators should begin the analysis section with a presentation of the comparative characteristics of the patients. Important characteristics to compare include the type, severity, and duration of the patient's medical condition, demographics, and use of concurrent medication. The investigators should briefly indicate (perhaps in tabular form) if the experimental and control patients are comparable and should discuss any statistically significant differences that are noted. When the experimental and control groups differ on known and important characteristics, their influence can be minimized through the use of a statistical technique known as analysis of covariance (ANCOVA). ANCOVA adjusts for the baseline differences among the trial groups and essentially removes the influence of these differences from the analysis of drug treatment effects. ANCOVA is a very useful technique for adjusting known differences among patients who have been randomly assigned to the experimental or control groups. It is less effective in those trials in which the patients were not randomly assigned.[1,16,22-25]

16. Were descriptive statistics used properly to describe the trial results?

After the raw data are collected, they should be organized into a useable form and the characteristics of patients and their responses should be numerically described. This process is often referred to as descriptive statistics and is intended to provide a convenient, effective method for the investigator to describe the reported results. Descriptive statistics involve classifying the data, examining the distribution of the data, providing measures of the group characteristics (central tendencies), and identifying the degree of variation of individual scores from the group score (variability).[6,26-28]

Investigators can use a wide variety of statistical methods to describe the data collected. Although the choice of method is usually left to the investigator, there are standard approaches that are recommended. Some of these approaches are described briefly in Table 17-3. Regardless of the approach, the potential for using the descriptive statistic in a misleading manner always exists. A flawed approach to describing the data can result in inappropriate conclusions and misleading theories about the data collected. [6,14,26,28]

Table 17-3. Selected Statistical Methods Used to Describe Data

Statistical method	Description
Classifying data	Classifying data into different categories or scales such as nominal, ordinal, interval or ratio
Assessing normality	Examining whether the data are arranged in a normal distribution through the use of frequency distributions, histograms, or scatter diagrams
Measuring centrality	Describing the central part of the data with measures such as the mean, median, or mode
Measuring variability	Estimating the spread of the data through the use of measures such as the range or standard deviation
Finding true scores	Using the confidence interval to determine the range of values that will contain the "true" score
Examining relationships	Using correlational analysis and linear regression to examine relationships between two or more measures

a.   Classifying data

Data collected regarding each patient's response to drug therapy can be classified into four different categories or scales: nominal, ordinal, interval, and ratio. The most useful are the interval or ratio scales.[6,28] Each classification is described in Table 17-4.

Table 17-4. Classification of Data Scales[6,28]

Classification	Description
Nominal	The least complicated scale and weakest level of measurement. Data are classified by an assigned number in which patients are placed in subgroups based on similar characteristics. Nominal scales are used to describe two or more groups of patients. Examples would include assigning numerical categories that designate patients as male or female, cured or not cured, or receiving the investigational or control drug. The numbers selected to describe each group are arbitrary and are usually chosen at the discretion of the investigator. There cannot be any overlap among the groups.
Ordinal	The data are ranked in a specific order, usually low to high. A typical ordinal scale would rank the amount of ankle swelling from "one" (very little or none) to "three" (a great deal). The numbers chosen are scored on a continuum, although the level of difference between different sets of numbers may not be consistent. The actual number assigned is not important as long as the different evaluators consistently assign higher (or lower) numbers to the relatively more important subgroup.
Interval	The scales are based on pre-determined numbering like ordinal scales but also include a consistent difference between each number. The scale lacks a true "zero point" that would indicate no data present. An example would be a measure of the patient's age.
Ratio	Similar to the interval scale except that there is a true zero point. Heart rate, blood pressure, and time to demonstrate an effect are examples of ratio scales.

Data can also be classified as continuous or discrete (or categorical). Continuous data scales provide the theoretical possibility of observing an infinite number of equally spaced values on a scale. Interval and ratio scales can be classified as continuous data scales. Conversely, discrete data scales have a finite number of values. Ordinal and nominal scales are examples of discrete data scales. In practice, the distinction between the two scales is often unclear because instruments generally measure a finite range of data. In addition, data based on continuous scales are often rescaled by the investigator into discrete categories.[23,29,30]

While the definition of the type of scales used to describe the data collected is standardized and often based on the type of measuring instrument used, the way in which investigators use the scales can vary. The choice of method can greatly affect the interpretation of the results. If an investigator converts continuously scaled data into discrete groups, valuable data may be lost. Any reclassification of the data should clearly distinguish between the different categories. An example would be the data collected to assess the efficacy of an investigational antihypertensive drug. The primary outcome assessed may be "blood pressure control", as measured by changes in the blood pressure. Although blood pressure is measured on a continuous scale, investigators will often divide the patients into subgroups who are "controlled" and "not controlled" with the former consisting of patients with a diastolic pressure lower than 95 mmHg on the sphygmomanometer. The investigator would report a percentage of patients who achieve the desired goal, but the results may be misleading. Some patients classified as "controlled" may have a diastolic blood pressure as high as 94 mmHg. That value is not very different from the minimum value of 95 mmHg needed to classify a patient as "not controlled".[3,6]

The type of data scales created by the investigator influences the choice of statistical tests used and their effectiveness in detecting differences between the experimental and control groups. The more powerful statistical tests should be used with only continuously scaled data. In addition, loss of information with the use of discrete scales makes any statistical test less sensitive in identifying true differences between the experimental and control groups (see question 18).[3,6,8,30]

b.   Assessing normality

Normal distribution of the data collected means that the data are spread symmetrically into a bell-shaped curve, which is sometimes called a Gaussian, normal distribution, or normal probability curve (Figure 17-1A). Most of the powerful statistical techniques are based on the assumption that the data are distributed normally. Normality of the data should be assessed in order to distinguish the distribution scheme from other less frequent (and undesirable) types of distributions such as bimodal curves, rectangular distribution, or skewed data curves (Figure 17-1B-1E). Bimodal distributions occur when the data are clustered around two high points in the curve (Figure 17-1B). An example would be a clinical drug trial for an analgesic in which most patients experience one of two responses: no effect or complete relief of pain. A rectangular distribution would show equal frequency of occurrence for all levels of a particular characteristic, such as a bioavailability trial in which the drug product is completely absorbed by all patients in the trial (Figure 17-1C). Skewed data curves occur when the data are distributed asymmetrically with one side of the curve extending out in an elongated fashion (Figures 17-1D and 1E).[23,28,29,31-34]

Figure 17-1.   Possible Distribution Curves for Data Collected in Clinical Drug Trials[a]

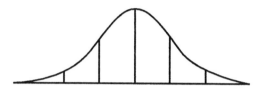

A. Gaussian or Normal Probability Curve

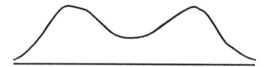

B. Bimodal Distribution Curve

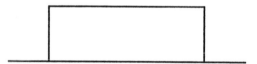

C. Rectangular Distribution Curve

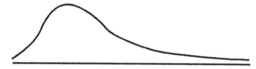 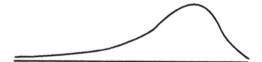

D & E. Skewed Data Curves

[a]   Adapted with permission from Figures 1 and 2 in Gaddis ML, Gaddis GM. Introduction to biostatistics: part 1, basic concepts. *Ann Emerg Med* 1990;19:86-89.

One of the easiest ways to examine normality is to prepare a table of frequency distributions which organizes the data into discrete intervals (Table 17-5). Methods vary for presenting frequency distributions in tables. Nevertheless, the intervals chosen should reflect the data collected and empty intervals or those with small numbers should be avoided. The number of intervals chosen should be sufficient to clearly describe the data, but an excessive number is undesirable.[23]

Table 17-5. An Example Table of Frequency Distribution: Serum Cholesterol Changes for 156 Patients after Administration of a Cholesterol Lowering Drug[a]

Interval (mg%)[b]	Frequency (patients)
-100 to -81	1
-80 to -61	6
-60 to -41	16
-40 to -21	31
-20 to -1	40
0 to +19	43
+20 to +39	16
+40 to +59	3

[a] Adapted with permission from Table 1.2 in Bolton S. Pharmaceutical statistics. 2nd ed. New York: Marcel Dekker, 1990:6.

[b] Represents the change from baseline in serum cholesterol after the cholesterol lowering drug was administered.

Another approach is to present data as cumulative frequencies which can be used to quickly demonstrate the cumulative effect of the investigational drug (Table 17-6). As indicated in Table 17-6, about 60% of the patients had their cholesterol reduced by the drug.

Table 17-6. An Example Table of Cumulative Frequency Distributions: Serum Cholesterol Changes for 156 Patients after Administration of a Cholesterol Lowering Drug[a]

Interval (mg%)[b]	Cumulative Frequency (patients)	Cumulative Proportion
-100 to -81	1	0.01
-80 to -61	7	0.04
-60 to -41	23	0.15
-40 to -21	54	0.35
-20 to -1	94	0.60
0 to +19	137	0.88
+20 to +39	153	0.98
+40 to +59	156	1.00

[a] Adapted with permission from Table 1.2 in Bolton S. Pharmaceutical statistics. 2nd ed. New York: Marcel Dekker, 1990:6.

[b] Represents the change from baseline in serum cholesterol after the cholesterol lowering drug was administered.

Graphic approaches to assessing normality are illustrated by histograms or scatter diagrams. Histograms are graphs in which the frequency of each patient response is represented by an area interval (Figure 17-2). Histograms can be considered graphical representations of frequency distributions and are subject to the same type of guidelines. Scatter diagrams are graphs that show the relationship between two continuously scaled measures (Figure 17-3). Histograms or scatter diagrams may provide better visual displays of data distribution than tables but lack the detail of the tabular method.[23,35,36]

Figure 17-2.   Sample Histogram Showing the Serum Cholesterol Changes for 156 Patients After Administration of a Cholesterol Lowering Drug[a,b]

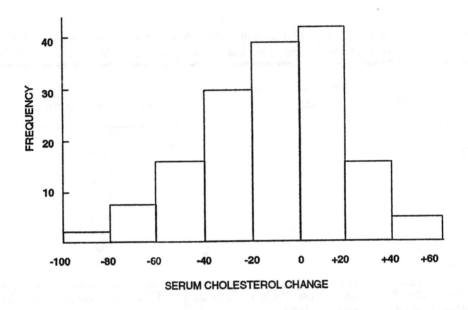

---

[a]   The horizontal axis represents the change from baseline in serum cholesterol after the cholesterol lowering drug is administered. The vertical axis represents the number of patients in each interval.

[b]   Adapted with permission from Figure 2.2 in Bolton S. Pharmaceutical statistics. 2nd ed. New York: Marcel Dekker, 1990:37.

Figure 17-3.   Sample Scatter Diagram Showing the Relationship Between Serum
Immunoglobulin E (IgE) and Age[a]

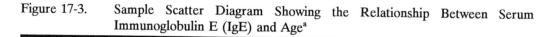

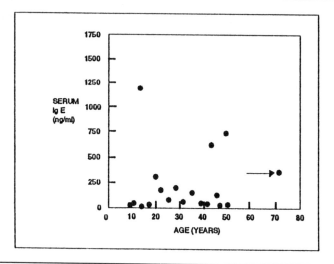

[a]   Adapted with permission from Figure 3.1 in O'Brien PC, Shampo MA. Statistics for
clinicians: 3. Graphic displays-scatter diagrams. *Mayo Clin Proc* 1981;56:196-7.

c.   Measuring centrality

Measures of centrality or central tendency include the mean, median, and mode and are
used to measure the central part of the data. The most common measure of centrality is
the mean, which is the arithmetic average of the data values. The mean is most effective
for normally distributed data that are ratio- or intervally-scaled. The measure is less
effective for ordinally-scaled data and is of little value for data that are nominally scaled.
The accuracy of the mean is distorted when extreme values, known as outliers, are present
in the data. The mean is also more likely to be distorted if there are relatively few patients
enrolled in the trial.[6,23,32]

The median is the middle value (the 50th percentile) of a set of data. Thus, half of the
data points are less than the median and half are greater. Unlike the mean, the median
is unaffected by outliers and may be better for data not normally distributed. The median
is a better measure than the mean for ordinally-scaled data but, like the mean, is not useful
for nominally-scaled data.[23,32,34]

The mode is the value that occurs most frequently in the data. The mode is used less often
than the mean or median and is useful with data that are clustered around two high points
(bimodal curve) or one relatively high peak. However, the mode is less useful than other
measures of centrality in data generated from small numbers of patients. Unlike the mean
and median, the mode can be used to describe nominally-scaled data.[23,32,37]

While measures of centrality tend to be effective even if some of the assumptions regarding the distribution or the scaling of the data are violated, the choice of which measures to use should be based on a clear understanding of how the data are distributed. Although the mean, median, or mode represent the same value when the data are normally distributed (Figure 17-4A), they are no longer interchangeable when the data distributions become skewed or bimodal (Figures 17-4B and 4C). Thus, use of the wrong descriptive statistic can result in a misleading assessment of the data and a distorted impression of the effectiveness of the investigational drug.[29,32,37]

Figure 17-4.   Comparison of the Mean, Median, and Mode with Different Distributions of Clinical Data[a]

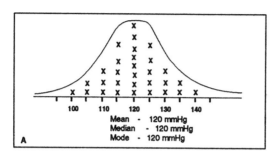

A. Mean, Median, and Mode for a Normal Distribution Curve Showing the Systolic Blood Pressures of Men Aged 31-40

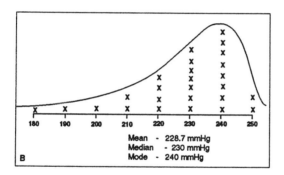

B. Mean, Median, and Mode for a Skewed Distribution Curve Showing the Systolic Blood Pressures of Patients with Renovascular Hypertension

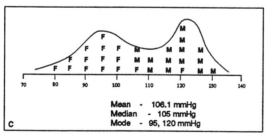

C. Mean, Median, and Mode for a Bimodal Distribution Curve Showing the Systolic Blood Pressures in Young Men and in Pregnant Women[b]

---

[a]   Adapted with permission from Figures 1 through 3 in Gaddis GM, Gaddis ML. Introduction to biostatistics: part 2, descriptive statistics. *Ann Emerg Med* 1990;19:309-15.

[b]   M denotes male subjects and F denotes female subjects

d.   Measuring variability

Regardless of which method is used to describe the center part of the data, other measures are needed to assess the variability or spread. Common measures of variability are the range, percentile, and standard deviation. The purpose of these measures is to determine how closely individual patient values cluster around the center part of the data. A large variability in the data suggests the presence of a flaw in the trial design: unreliable measures may have been used, the subjects selected may not be very similar, or the data collected may not be normally distributed. The last problem would make the use of many of the descriptive statistics and tests of significance less appropriate (see Question 18).[23,29,32,34]

The range is the difference between the smallest and largest value in the data set. Although easy to understand, the range has limited use because it is strongly influenced by the most extreme values in the data and tends to be affected by the number of patients in the trial, increasing with the size of the sample. The range should be used only as a rough measure of the variability.[23,29,32,34]

Percentiles are measures of variability that are based on the median value, which would be considered the 50th percentile of the range of data in a clinical drug trial. The most likely use of percentiles is through the use of the interquartile range, which is the interval between the data score at the first quartile (25th percentile) and the third quartile (75th percentile). The interquartile range is used to get a rough impression of the middle 50% of the data and has an advantage over other measures of variability because it is less dependent on the number of patients enrolled. Another advantage is that the assumption of a normal distribution is not needed.[23,29,30,32,34]

The standard deviation (SD) is the most commonly used measure of variability. If all patient data scores were the same as the group mean, the standard deviation would be zero. Conversely, the standard deviation would increase as the patient data scores are further from the group mean. The standard deviation is commonly expressed as the "mean +/- SD". An example would be the reporting of the mean serum theophylline levels of a group of patients as 14.2 +/- 2.9 µg/ml. The utility of the standard deviation is based on its ability to more accurately define the distribution of the data than the other measures of variability. Assuming that the data are distributed normally, it is expected that 68.2% of the data scores would lie one standard deviation on either side of the mean and 95.4% of the scores would occur within two standard deviations. Almost all the values (99.7%) would be within three standard deviations of the mean (Figure 17-5). Thus, a mean serum theophylline level of 14.2 +/- 2.9 µg/ml means that 68.2% of the patients had serum levels between 11.3 and 17.1 µg/ml, 95.4% had levels between 8.4 and 20.0 µg/ml, and 99.7% had levels between 5.5 and 22.9 µg/ml. A measure closely related to the standard deviation is the variance, which is a more general measure of the spread of the data. The variance is the square of the standard deviation.[5,6,29,32,34]

Figure 17-5.   Use of the Standard Deviation in a Normal Distribution: Theoretical Curve of Plasma Drug Levels Attained One Hour After Oral Administration of 650 mg of Acetaminophen[a]

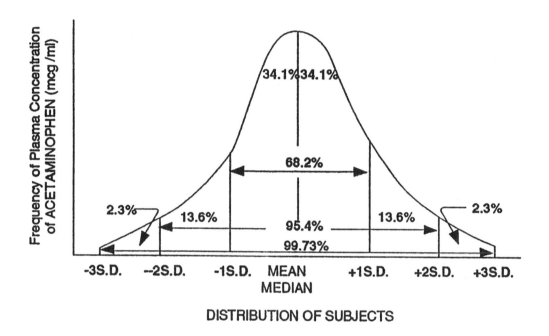

a   Adapted with permission from Figure 1 in Bennett RW, Popovich NG. Statistical inference as applied to bioavailability data--a guide for the practicing pharmacists. *Am J Hosp Pharm* 1977;34:712-23.

A measure that is often confused with the standard deviation is the standard error of the mean or SEM. This measure is sometimes called the standard deviation of the mean. The standard error of the mean is based on the premise that each sample obtained from the target population would have a group mean that differs from the "true" or population mean. The degree of variation that occurs each time a patient sample is obtained is measured by the standard error of the mean. Less variation suggests that each group sample mean obtained is close to the population mean and would produce more applicable results. The standard error of the mean is derived from the standard deviation and is always smaller, which sometimes results in misleading use of the statistic. Some investigators erroneously use the standard error of the mean as a measure of variability in order to give the impression that less variation is present in the data.[3,6,15,23,30,32,38]

e. Finding true scores

Confidence intervals (CIs) are used to find the "true" score of a statistic by estimating the range of scores in which the true value is likely to occur. Confidence limits represent the upper and lower extent of the confidence interval. A confidence interval can be created for a variety of statistics such as the population group mean, median values, and response rates to the investigational drug. The accepted width of the confidence interval depends on the variability of the data and an arbitrarily chosen degree of confidence, traditionally 95%. For example, the confidence interval of the mean serum level of acetaminophen obtained one hour after administration might be reported as 6.0 µg/ml with a 95% confidence interval of 1.5 µg/ml. Thus, the results indicate that a 95% probability exists that the serum acetaminophen level in other samples of patients tested under the same conditions will be between 3.0 and 9.0 µg/ml. Confidence intervals can be used to quickly compare the experimental and control groups or to assess the reliability of the measurement process. Like other estimates of variability, narrower confidence intervals indicate that a more homogeneous group of patients was enrolled in the clinical drug trial or that more reliable measures were used to collect the data.[30,32,37]

f. Examining relationships

Investigators are often interested in exploring the strength of relationships between various measures used in the clinical drug trial in order to minimize the influence of factors other than the investigational drug on the efficacy and safety measures used. Two common methods used for assessing relationships are correlational analysis and linear regression.

The purpose of correlational analysis is to evaluate the strength and direction of a relationship between two or more measures. An example would be the examination of the relationship between the patient's age, weight, height and the investigational drug's serum level. The measures most often used in correlational analysis are the Pearson product moment correlation and Spearman rank order correlation which are represented by the notation r. Pearson or Spearman r values range from 0 (no association) to 1 (complete agreement). A minus sign is usually attached when the relationship is negative (i.e., going in an opposite direction). Because complete agreement between two measures is rare, the importance of any relationship is usually based on the subjective opinion of the investigators. Nevertheless, a relationship with a r value of 0.88 (normally reported as r = 0.88) between the patient's age and the investigational drug's serum level would generally be considered strong while a r value of 0.12 (reported as r = 0.12) would usually be considered weak. Correlational analysis should be limited only to the exploration of possible relationships among the measures present in the clinical drug trial because it tends to identify associations which are arbitrary and ambiguous. It should not be used to identify causal relationships.[6,33,39,40]

Linear regression describes the relationship between multiple measures by finding the best fitting straight line among the data collected. Mathematically, linear regression examines the rate of change in one measure that is related to a change in another and is expressed by the following formula: $y = a + bx + e$. The letter *y* represents one measure and *x* is the other. The notation *a* is the y intercept or the point on the y axis where the regression lines cross (the value of y when x = 0), *b* is the slope or the amount of change in y for every unit increase in x, and *e* is the term for the random error present in the data. The random error term is often eliminated from the equation.

Simple linear regression is used to examine the relationship between two measures and multiple linear regression explores the association among more than two measures. The regression line is usually calculated with the least squares method, which is designed to find where the line comes closest to running through all the data points (best fit). The most commonly used measure of the effectiveness of the linear regression line is the coefficient of determination, which is represented by the notation r^2. The r^2 is equal to 1 when all the data points are on the regression line and is equal to 0 when there is no linear relationship among the data. Like the r term in correlational analysis, the r^2 is rarely equal to 1. Thus, the importance of the r^2 of any linear regression is based on the investigator's subjective opinion. Linear regression, like correlational analysis, should be limited to examining associations among the various measures in the clinical drug trial but should not be used as the sole basis for establishing a causal relationship between two or more measures.[6,23,39,41]

17. Were figures, graphs, or tables used properly to present the trial results?

One of the most important objectives of the analysis section is to present the data clearly and concisely through a combination of figures, graphs, tables, or text. Because there are no uniform guidelines on how to present data, the approaches vary, depending on the preferences of the investigator or the publisher. Some investigators prefer to present results graphically, while others favor the greater detail that can be provided in tables or text. Various publishers of scientific journals encourage use of the graphs or tables, while others restrict the use of either because of space limitations. Regardless of the technique used, the number of figures, graphs, or tables should be restricted to that sufficient to complement each other and the text in explaining results and supporting the investigator's observations and conclusions. An excessive number of figures, graphs, or tables can unnecessarily fragment the analysis and create a cluttered image. Redundancy should be avoided.[5,14,16]

a. Use of tables

Tables are useful to present numerical data that would require several long and awkward sentences to describe. Several techniques are recommended in Table 17-7 to ensure that the results are presented clearly in tables.[14,16,42,43]

Table 17-7. Techniques for Displaying Numbers in Tables[14,43]

Techniques	Description
Use of digits	Use as few as possible (0.11 vs 0.1105)
Columns and rows	Present vertically in columns rather than horizontally in rows
Margins	Margin and row averages should be reported
Order	Place in consistent, logical order such as decreasing or increasing importance
Clarity	Use layout to ensure clarity and to make information presented self-explanatory
Summaries	Text summaries of the tables should be brief and focus on the main points of the tables

Tables 17-8 and 17-9 illustrate how the guidelines can be applied to make a table easier to read. The tables compare the death rates observed in four groups in which anesthetics were used in surgeries with high death rates. Table 17-8 presents data in a manner which ignored the guidelines presented in Table 17-7. The table appears cluttered and difficult to read. The use of five digit figures and horizontal presentation of important categories confuses the reader.

Table 17-8. An Example Table Which Lacks Clarity: Death Rates in Proportions for High Death Rate Operations by Anesthetic Risk Levels[a]

Anesthetic Risk Code	Halothane	Nitrous Oxide	Cyclo-propane	Ether	Other
Unknown	0.11369	0.08682	0.08147	0.06148	0.09957
Risk 1	0.02454	0.02452	0.01634	0.01355	0.03358
Risk 2	0.05471	0.06893	0.04941	0.03812	0.05859
Risk 3	0.12471	0.16599	0.18187	0.11453	0.15306
Risk 4	0.15892	0.23140	0.18582	0.17919	0.35531
Risk 5	0.04665	0.06759	0.05725	0.04898	0.07606
Risk 6	0.22143	0.12996	0.17615	0.16008	0.17741
Risk 7	0.44164	0.43689	0.36689	0.62121	0.43348

[a]   Adapted with permission from Table 1 in Bailar JC, Mosteller F. Guidelines for statistical reporting in articles for medical journals. In Bailar JC and Mosteller F, eds. Medical use of statistics. Boston: NEJM books 1992:325.

Table 17-9 illustrates the results organized according to the guidelines of Table 17-7. The number of digits has been reduced to one or two, the major categories of numbers are presented vertically, marginal and row averages are provided, and the order is based on the weighted average in the last column.

Table 17-9. An Example Table based on Clarity Guidelines: Death Rates in Percentages for High Death Rate Operations by Anesthetic Risk Levels Versus Anesthetic Risk[a]

Anesthetic Group	Anesthetic Risk Code								
	1	2	5	UNK	3	6	4	7	WA
Other	3	6	8	10	15	18	36	43	11.7
Nitrous oxide	2	7	7	9	17	13	23	44	10.3
Cyclo-propane	2	5	6	8	18	18	19	37	9.8
Halothane	2	5	5	11	12	22	16	44	8.7
Ether	1	4	5	6	11	16	18	62	6.1
WA	2.2	5.5	5.7	9.6	14.6	17.4	20.6	42.4	9.3

UNK = unknown   WA = weighted average

[a] Adapted with permission from Table 2 in Bailar JC, Mosteller F. Guidelines for statistical reporting in articles for medical journals. In Bailar JC and Mosteller F, eds. Medical use of statistics. Boston: NEJM books 1992:327.

Table 17-9 should be summarized in the following manner:[14]

> "The table shows that the overall weighted percentage of deaths in these high death rate operations is 9.3%. When the risk levels are arranged according to the average death rate for the risk, each anesthetic leads to a nearly monotonic increase in death rate according to risk, the order being codes 1,2,5, unknown, 3,6,4, and 7. The last five groups have sharply higher death rates with Risk 7 (moribund) giving 42.4% . . . the death rates do not change much from one anesthetic group to another. . . . In the low-risk code (1,2,5, Unknown) patients, halothane, cyclopropane, and nitrous oxide have very similar rates for these high death operations."

b.   Contingency tables

A contingency table is an important tabular tool to present relationships between categories of information such as analgesic pain relief (yes/no) categorized by gender (male/female).

An N x N contingency table would be formed to illustrate the relationship where N equaled the number of categories (Table 17-10). The display of the data in the table is sometimes called a cross tabulation. Table 17-10 represents a cross tabulation of pain relief and gender.[44]

Table 17-10.   A 2 x 2 Contingency Table Showing the Relationship Between Pain Relief and Gender

| Gender | Pain Relief | | Totals |
	Yes	No	
Male	88 (44%)	112 (56%)	200 (67%)
Female	60 (60%)	40 (40%)	100 (33%)
Totals	148 (49%)	152 (51%)	300 (100%)

The objective of contingency table analysis is to identify possible differences in responses when patients are divided into subgroups. In Table 17-10, the contingency table is used to determine if the response to the analgesic would be different in males versus females. According to the table, a difference may exist because a higher percentage of females (60%) than males (44%) reported pain relief. This difference should be examined statistically with a significance test such as Chi square or Fisher's exact test to ensure that it is not a chance occurrence (see Question 18).

A possible danger of contingency table analysis is the identification of subgroup differences that may not be important. An example is a phenomenon known as Simpson's paradox. In this phenomenon, differences noted when patients are divided into subgroups disappear when the subgroups are combined. Simpson's paradox occurs when there is a stronger relationship between the characteristics in the subgroup than in the group as a whole. Using the data shown in Table 17-10, Simpson's paradox may occur if significantly more men were assigned to the experimental rather than the control group. Thus, the patients in the experimental group (who would be predominantly male) would be less responsive to the analgesic drugs used in the clinical drug trial than the group of control patients (see Question 18).

c.   Figures or graphs

The purpose of a figure or graph is to present a quick, easy to understand, visual impression of the reported results. While such displays do not provide the detail found in tables or text, figures or graphs can clarify or reinforce conclusions based on the results presented in the tables or text of a research report. In addition, graphical displays tend to be more effective than tables or text at drawing attention to important characteristics of the data presented. Several helpful guidelines should be followed to ensure that figures and graphs are used properly (Table 17-11). Like tables, figures and graphs should be clear enough to be self-explanatory and not dependent on related information provided in the text of the research report.[3,23,35,36]

Table 17-11. Guidelines for Proper Use of Figures and Graphs.[23]

Guideline	Description
Title	Clear and brief description of what the graphic display depicts
Axes	Horizontal and vertical axes should be clearly defined and labeled Zero points of both axes should be provided if appropriate
Spacing of data	The numbers assigned to each axis should be appropriately spaced to cover the range of data collected for the clinical drug trial
Excluding data	"Broken" lines should be used to clearly indicate if a range of data or specific data "outliers" are not included in the axis
Symbols	Symbols used in the graphic display need to be explained clearly
Source of data	The source of the data should be clearly described including the numbers of patients or observations which contributed to the display
Differentiating data curves	An easily understood method (such as different symbols) of distinguishing data curves must be used when two or more curves are displayed
Standard deviations	Should be included where appropriate to demonstrate the variability of the data

d.   Graphical display of data

Some of the methods used to graphically display the data are histograms, scatter diagrams, frequency polygons, cumulative distribution polygons, pie charts or survival curves (Table 17-12). The choice of which method to use is usually based on the type of data to be displayed.[3,23,35,36]

Table 17-12.   Types of Figures and Graphs Used to Display Data

Figure or Graph	Description
Histogram (bar graph)	Presents patient responses in intervals represented by bars
Scatter diagram (plot)	Displays the distribution of data (individual scores) for two or more measures
Frequency polygon	Displays the distribution of data (ranges or intervals) for two or more measures
Cumulative distribution polygon	Shows the cumulative effect of a measure
Pie chart	Displays categorical data
Survival curve	Displays the probability of survival from a disease if left untreated

1)   Histogram or bar graph

Histograms or bar graphs are most effective in displaying information if the intervals are of equal width (histogram A, Figure 17-6). Interpretation of the histogram becomes more difficult when the intervals are not of equal length (histogram B, Figure 17-6). In addition, the horizontal axis of a histogram should be marked at regular, unbroken intervals and the vertical axis should start at zero in order to clearly display the distribution of the data. Histograms with irregular intervals could distort the differences between the experimental and control groups. The intervals chosen should reflect the data collected and intervals containing small numbers should be avoided.[3,23,35]

Figure 17-6.   Sample Histograms Showing the Serum Cholesterol Changes for 156 Patients after Administration of a Cholesterol Lowering Drug[a]

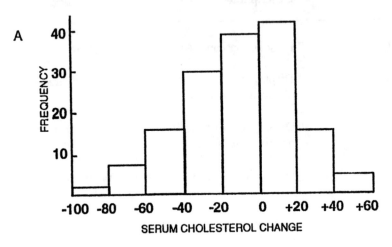

A. Serum Cholesterol Changes Shown with Intervals of Equal Length[b]

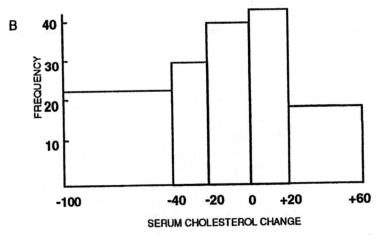

B. Serum Cholesterol Changes Shown with Intervals of Unequal Length[b]

---

[a]   Adapted with permission from Figure 2.2 in Bolton S. Pharmaceutical statistics. 2nd ed. New York: Marcel Dekker, 1990:37.

[b]   The horizontal axis represents the change from baseline in serum cholesterol after the cholesterol lowering drug is administered. The vertical axis represents the number of patients in each interval.

2)   Scatter diagram or plot

Scatter diagrams or plots are designed to demonstrate the relationship between two measures such as the association between the mean plasma level of acetaminophen and length of time after administration (Figure 17-7). As shown in Figure 17-7, the mean plasma level peaks at about 90 minutes after administration then gradually decreases. Scatter diagrams are useful for displaying the variability of the data, especially when there are relatively few data points collected in the trial.[23,36,37]

Figure 17-7.   An Example Scatter Diagram that Shows the Mean Concentration of Acetaminophen versus Administration Time for Two Products[a]

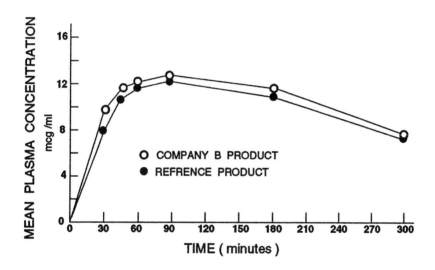

[a]   Adapted with permission from Figure 4 in Bennett RW, Popovich NG. Statistical inference as applied to bioavailability data-a guide for the practicing pharmacists. *Am J Hosp Pharm* 1977;34:712-23.

3) Frequency polygon

Frequency polygons are similar to scatter diagrams and are designed to compare two types of data on the same graph (Figure 17-8). The major difference from scatter diagrams is the use of intervals as connecting points rather than individual data scores. Frequency polygons can be used for larger sets of data than scatter diagrams. In Figure 17-8, the frequency polygon indicates that girls as a group tend to have higher levels of serum triglycerides than boys.[35]

Figure 17-8.   Sample Frequency Polygon Comparing the Serum Triglycerides Levels of 96 Boys and 64 Girls[a]

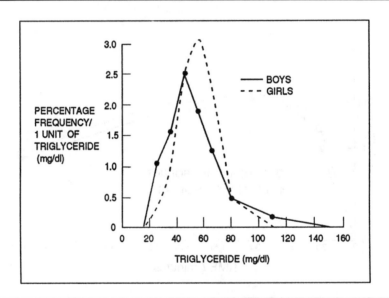

[a]   Adapted with permission from Figure 2.3 in O'Brien PC, Shampo MA. Statistics for clinicians: 2. Graphic displays-histograms, frequency polygons, and cumulative distribution polygons. *Mayo Clin Proc* 1981;56:126-8.

4) Cumulative distribution polygon

Cumulative distribution polygons are similar to cumulative frequency tables and are useful for quickly establishing the percentage of patients at or below a certain level. Using some of the data shown in Figure 17-8, the cumulative distribution polygon shown in Figure 17-9 indicates that most of the boys (88%) have serum triglyceride levels of 80 mg/dl or less.[35]

Figure 17-9.   Sample Cumulative Distribution Polygon Showing the Serum Triglycerides
                Levels of 96 Boys[a]

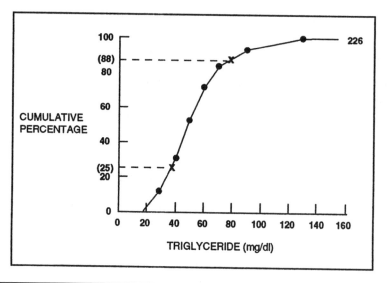

[a]   Adapted with permission from Figure 2.4 in O'Brien PC, Shampo MA. Statistics for
clinicians: 2. Graphic displays--histograms, frequency polygons, and cumulative distribution
polygons. *Mayo Clin Proc* 1981;56:126-8.

5) Pie chart

Pie charts provide a useful method of displaying categorical data such as percentages of male/female, cure/no cure, and response levels of good, fair, and poor (Figure 17-10). Pie charts are most effective when providing an overview of the results. Although easy to understand, pie charts need to be constructed carefully. Use of a large number of categories can be confusing and segments that are about the same size are difficult to distinguish from each other. The pie chart in Figure 17-10 represents the proportion of patients with good, fair, or poor responses to an investigational drug. The chart clearly indicates that most of the patients responded positively to the investigational drug but also highlights the percentage of poor responders by partially "removing" the section from the pie chart.[23]

Figure 17-10.   Sample Pie Chart Categorizing Patient Responses to a Drug in a Clinical Trial[a]

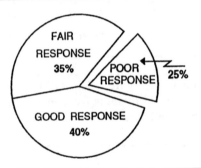

a   Adapted with permission from Figure 2.17 in Bolton S. Pharmaceutical statistics. 2nd ed. New York: Marcel Dekker, 1990:54.

6) Survival curve

The approach to displaying the survival experience for a group of patients is usually called a survival curve. Survival curves estimate the likelihood of survival for a group of patients and are especially useful in studies of life-threatening illnesses such as acquired immunodeficiency syndrome (AIDS) or various forms of cancer. A common type of survival curve is called the Kaplan-Meier estimated survival curve (Figure 17-11). The curve in Figure 17-11 compares the likelihood of survival for a group of patients diagnosed with lymphoma and presenting clinical symptoms. The horizontal axis represents the time since diagnosis while the vertical axis represents the probability of survival. According to the figure, 60% of patients suffering from clinical symptoms of lymphoma survive at least one year but less than 40% survive for three or more years following diagnosis. The data presented in the curve would be graphically compared with data obtained from patients enrolled in a clinical drug trial for an investigational drug designed to treat lymphoma. The investigational drug would be considered effective if the survival rate of the patients in the experimental group was higher than the expected rate illustrated by the survival curve.[33,38]

Figure 17-11.   Sample Survival Curve for 31 Patients Diagnosed with Lymphoma and Presenting with Clinical Symptoms[a]

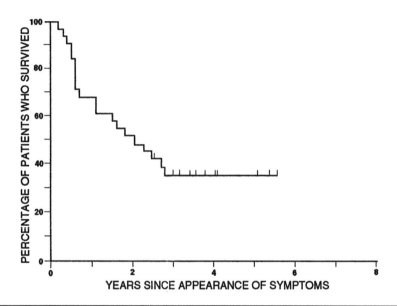

[a]   Adapted with permission from Figure 6.1 in Matthews DE, Farwell VT. Using and understanding medical statistics. 2nd ed. Basel, Switzerland: S. Karger AG, 1988:68.

e.   Identifying misleading graphical displays of data

Graphic displays can present results in a misleading manner. One misleading approach is to manipulate the horizontal and vertical axis to show that one drug is superior to another. This is illustrated by the bar graphs shown in Figure 17-12. In bar graph A, the effect of the bronchodilators, epinephrine and terbutaline, on heart rate appears to be similar. However, altering the vertical axis as indicated in bar graph B gives the visual impression that epinephrine decreases the heart rate much more than terbutaline.[45]

Figure 17-12.   Examples of Misleading Bar Graphs[a,b] Showing the Mean Heart Rate Before and After Treatment with Epinephrine or Terbutaline[c]

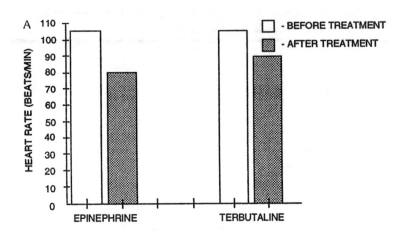

[a]   Bar graph A depicts changes in heart rate after the administration of epinephrine or terbutaline using a scale with a range of 0 to 110 beats per minute.

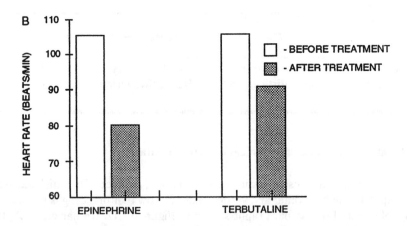

[b]   Bar graph B depicts changes in heart rate after the administration of epinephrine or terbutaline using a scale with a range of 60 to 110 beats per minute.

[c]   Adapted with permission from Figure 1 in Elenbaas JK, Cuddy PG, Elenbaas RM. Evaluating the medical literature part III: results and discussion. *Ann Emerg Med* 1983;12:679-686.

Graphic displays can be misleading when the data selected for illustration are incomplete. The problem is illustrated by a clinical drug trial in which two bronchodilators, epinephrine and terbutaline, were compared. Data from the trial are shown in Table 17-13 and represent the forced expiratory volumes (FEVs) of patients before and after administration of the bronchodilators.

Table 17-13.   Comparative Forced Expiratory Volumes (FEVs) of Epinephrine and Terbutaline (N = 50)[a]

	Epinephrine		Terbutaline	
Administration Time	FEV[b]	Change[c]	FEV[b]	Change[c]
Baseline	1.25		1.80	
20 minutes	1.50	0.25 (20)	2.05	0.25 (14)
60 minutes	2.50	1.25 (100)	3.05	1.25 (69)

[a]   Modified from Table 2 in Elenbaas JK, Cuddy PG, Elenbaas RM. Evaluating the medical literature part III: results and discussion. *Ann Emerg Med* 1983;12:679-686.
[b]   The forced expiratory volume expressed in liters.
[c]   Represents change from baseline values. Percentage change is in parentheses.

Table 17-13 shows that the baseline FEV values of patients who received epinephrine were lower than those of patients who received terbutaline. The actual change in FEV was the same for both groups, although the mean 60-minute value for patients who received terbutaline was higher than for patients who received epinephrine. Because of the different baseline scores, the percentage change of FEV for terbutaline was less than that of epinephrine. Thus, graphic emphasis of only one part of the results could lead to a misleading conclusion. The misrepresentation is shown in Figures 17-13A-13C. Figure 17-13A shows the FEV at each measurement time. Because patients who received epinephrine had lower FEV values at baseline, it appears that epinephrine is inferior to terbutaline. The opposite impression occurs with Figure 17-13B. In this figure, percentage change was graphically displayed. The lower baseline values of patients receiving epinephrine create a greater percentage change, suggesting visually that epinephrine is superior to terbutaline. An appropriate graphic display is Figure 17-13C, where the actual change in FEV for both patient groups is shown. The graphs in Figure 17-13C can be displayed separately or combined in one graph. As indicated in the figures, the actual effects of epinephrine or terbutaline on FEV are identical.[45]

Figure 17-13.   Examples of Misleading Line Graphs Showing the Mean Forced Expiratory Volume (FEV) Before and After Treatment with Epinephrine or Terbutaline[a]

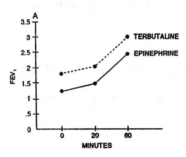

A.   Unadjusted FEV levels at each Measurement Time after the Administration of Epinephrine or Terbutaline

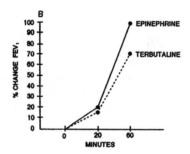

B.   Percent changes in FEV after the Administration of Epinephrine or Terbutaline

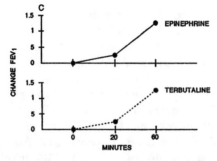

C.   Actual changes in FEV after the Administration of Epinephrine or Terbutaline

[a]   Adapted with permission from Figure 2 in Elenbaas JK, Cuddy PG, Elenbaas RM. Evaluating the medical literature part III: results and discussion. *Ann Emerg Med* 1983;12:679-686.

18. Was the approach described by the investigators appropriate for analyzing possible differences between the experimental and control groups?

The primary purpose of performing a clinical drug trial is to determine whether an investigational drug is superior in efficacy and safety to existing treatment for a particular disorder. From a statistical standpoint, this approach involves the process of inference, in which conclusions are derived from imperfect or incomplete data. Proper use of inferential statistics, also known as inductive statistics, involves adhering to a set of guidelines for data analysis (Table 17-14).[2,6,26,27]

Table 17-14.   Guidelines for Analyzing Differences between Experimental and Control Groups in a Clinical Drug Trial

Guidelines	Description
Develop hypotheses	Statistical tests need hypotheses developed prior to the research in order to properly examine differences between the experimental and control groups
Avoid Type I and Type II errors	False conclusions about the differences between the experimental and control groups need to be avoided
Proper choice of statistical tests	The most powerful statistical tests should be selected without making incorrect assumptions regarding the data to be analyzed
Planned statistical analysis	The differences to be examined need to be planned prior to the research and should be few in number in order to avoid the possibility of detecting chance differences

a.   Develop hypotheses

Inferential statistics involves using tests designed to limit the possibility that the differences observed between the experimental and control groups are due to a chance occurrence and not because of the investigational drug. Statistical testing usually involves the establishment of a hypothesis, which contains a quantitative statement about an effect. The hypothesis is usually stated in positive terms. An example would be the hypothesis that the antibiotic amoxicillin would cause a larger percentage reduction in the symptoms and signs of a urinary tract infection in an experimental group than treatment administered to a control group.   This hypothesis is typically known as the research or alternate hypothesis (sometimes designated as H_1).   Also established is the null or statistical hypothesis (sometimes designated as H_o), which is derived from the research hypothesis.   In the amoxicillin example, the null hypothesis would be that there are no differences between the experimental group receiving amoxicillin and the control group receiving another treatment.[26,37,46]

The null hypothesis, rather than the research hypothesis, is tested statistically because it is mathematically less complex. Only one type of difference can occur with the null hypothesis (no difference) while a wide range of differences can occur with the research hypothesis. Nevertheless, the null hypothesis and the research hypothesis are roughly opposite of each other. Thus, if the null hypothesis is "accepted", the research hypothesis must be "rejected". In contrast, the rejection of the null hypothesis does not necessarily mean that the research hypothesis is true because of the infinite range of possible alternate hypotheses besides those stated by the investigator. The typical null hypothesis for a clinical drug trial is that an investigational drug is not different than the control drug in efficacy and safety. The investigators' usual research hypothesis is that the investigational drug is superior. However, another set of research hypotheses could be that the investigational drug is inferior to the control drug in efficacy, safety, or both. Rejection of the null hypothesis indicates that a significant difference exists between the experimental and control group and that the difference between the groups is not due to chance alone.[47]

One of the most important issues in developing hypotheses is whether they were developed before or after the research began. Hypotheses developed before the research was started are known as *a priori* hypotheses and hypotheses developed after the data are collected are known as *post hoc* or *post priori* hypotheses. *Post hoc* hypotheses usually involve fitting data to a particular significance test rather than matching the test with the data. It is wise to regard any conclusions based on *post hoc* hypotheses cautiously. These conclusions are more likely to be based on chance occurrence than those based on the original hypothesis. Unplanned statistical analyses or *post hoc* analyses are sometimes referred to as "data dredging" or "data snooping" and should be viewed as the basis for future confirmatory research rather than as facts. Investigators should be candid in describing what part of their analysis was planned and which was not planned.[2,6,18,37,48]

b.   Avoid Type I and Type II errors

The rejection or acceptance of the null hypothesis is not made with absolute certainty. Two types of interpretive errors are possible. The Type I or alpha error occurs when the investigator concludes that an actual difference existed between the experimental and control groups when, in fact, it did not. This is also known as falsely rejecting the null hypothesis of no difference. Type II or beta error occurs when the investigator concludes that no difference existed between the trial groups when, in fact, it did. This error is also known as falsely accepting the null hypothesis of no difference. Type I and Type II errors are directly related. An increase in Type I error probability will result in a decrease in Type II error probability if other design factors are constant. The probability of making a Type I or alpha error is represented by the p value. Statistical significance is traditionally set at a p value of 0.05 (i.e. $p < 0.05$) which means that the investigator is 95% confident that a Type I error was not made. Investigators usually focus on statistical tests which examine the likelihood of a Type I error occurring and frequently do not assess the probability that a Type II error will occur. However, ignoring Type II errors would be a serious oversight because undetected, but "actual", differences may have importance in the clinical practice setting or because further evaluation of a promising investigational drug may seem unwarranted (see Question 20).[6,25,32,37,38,50,51]

c. Proper choice of statistical tests

1) tests of statistical significance

A wide variety of tests are available for determining whether the null hypothesis is true. These tests are often called tests of significance. The choice of which test to use is based on the characteristics of the data collected. The objective would be to select the most effective test for detecting true differences between the experimental and control groups. Choosing the proper test to use should be made before the trial begins, but changes can occur after reviewing the distribution of the data or after preliminary analysis. The effect of using the wrong type of significance test depends partially on the magnitude of the difference between the experimental and control groups. The choice of tests is less important if the different tests give essentially the same result. The selection of the proper test is important, however, where there is a strong likelihood that different results will occur depending on the test used. Thus, investigators may choose to report or emphasize only those statistical tests which support their hypotheses.[6,52,53]

2) parametric versus nonparametric tests

Based on the characteristics of the data collected, significance tests can be divided into parametric and nonparametric tests. Parametric tests require specific assumptions about the data collected (Table 17-15). Nonparametric tests are recommended if the distribution of data is unknown or the data do not meet the criteria necessary for parametric tests. Parametric tests are more powerful than nonparametric tests in identifying "real" differences between the experimental and control groups.[6,46,48,52-54]

Table 17-15.   Assumptions Required for the Use of Parametric Tests of Significance

- data collected are normally distributed
- variability of the data collected from the experimental and control group is roughly equal
- measures of patient response are independent and not related in any manner
- data are continuous with interval or ratio scales

3) parametric tests

The most commonly used parametric tests are the student t test and analysis of variance. A less commonly used test is the z test. The student t test (commonly referred to as the t test) is the suggested approach when the investigator is making a single comparison between the experimental and control group. Although the assumptions discussed in Table 17-15 are required for the t test, the test is still effective when these assumptions are not met in the strict sense. The only assumption that cannot be violated is the use of measures that are dependent on each other (e.g., studies for which baseline measures of the patient are compared to post-test measures). The presence of dependent measures would necessitate the use of a paired t test but the data would still need to meet the other assumptions of the t test. The paired t test assumes that the mean for one set of data is closely related to the other set of data. An example would be measures of the same patient's blood pressure taken at the beginning and end of a clinical drug trial.[6,47,51-52]

Like the t test, the z or critical ratio test assesses the difference between the means of the experimental and control groups. The z test is not used as often as the t test because it requires a less commonly occurring distribution of the data (standardized normal distribution) than the t test (student t distribution). In addition, the z test is less effective in testing the mean scores of a relatively small number of patients.[25,33,38]

The accepted method of analysis for comparing three or more groups is analysis of variance (ANOVA), which has a number of advantages over the use of multiple t tests (Table 17-16). Because it is exactly the same as the t test, ANOVA is rarely used for the comparison of two groups. ANOVA compares the variability of the subjects within each group to each other and to subjects in the other trial groups. Like the t test, ANOVA is effective even if most of the assumptions for parametric tests are not strictly met, with the exception of the assumption of independent measures.[6,31,48,55,56]

Table 17-16.   Advantages of Analysis of Variance Compared to Multiple t Tests

Advantage	Description
Probability of Type I error	Reduced likelihood of making a Type I error as the number of comparisons increases
Calculation	Less cumbersome to calculate
Detection	More powerful in detecting group differences
Examining independent effects	One type of ANOVA (factorial) can analyze different effects without increasing the chance of a Type I error occurring

The ANOVA procedure is limited to determining the probability that nonchance differences occurred among any of the treatment groups. The specific differences and the extent of these differences are determined by another set of related statistical tests. The tests are collectively called multiple comparison tests and are available in various forms such as the Least Significant Difference (LSD), Duncan's Multiple Range test, Nueman-Keuls test, Tukey's Multiple Range test, Bonferroni t procedure, and the Scheffe' procedure. All of the comparison tests are based on the t test but include corrections for the multiple comparisons being made and the increased likelihood of identifying "false" differences. The tests vary in how conservative they are in detecting differences. The choice of which test to use is usually based on the investigator's concern about the negative consequences of making either Type I or Type II errors.[6,23,25,48,55]

ANOVA designs vary in their complexity. The least complicated approach is one-way ANOVA. A typical one-way ANOVA design for a clinical drug trial would be to compare three different drug treatments in different trial groups but at the equivalent dose schedule. A more complex approach would be two-way ANOVA which would allow for the assessment of the effects of each drug treatment as well as for different dose levels. Another type of ANOVA, referred to as analysis of covariance (ANCOVA), is used to adjust for important baseline differences among the trial groups. The purpose of ANCOVA is to remove the influence of these differences from the analysis of the reported results. Other more complex ANOVA designs not typically used in clinical drug trials are hierarchical and split-plot factorial ANOVAs.[23,25,55,56]

4)   nonparametric tests

Nonparametric tests are useful when the characteristics of the data collected are not known or thought not to meet the assumptions required for use of parametric tests. The most commonly used nonparametric tests are listed in Table 17-17. As indicated in the table, the tests vary by the type of data they analyze (e.g., nominal, ordinal, interval, or ratio), the number of groups compared (two or greater than two), and whether the data were collected from paired (same patient) or independent (different patient) measures. The most commonly used nonparametric test is the Chi square, primarily because of its ease of use and comprehension.[31,38,47,50,54]

Table 17-17.   Description of Nonparametric Tests

Nonparametric test (groups)	Conditions for use
Chi square (2)	Nominal data, sample size >20, independent measures
Fisher's exact (2)	Nominal data, sample size 20 or less, independent measures
McNemar's (2)	Nominal data, paired measures
Mann-Whitney U (2) (Wilcoxon test)	Ordinal, interval, or ratio data not meeting t test assumptions and not grouped as cumulative frequencies, independent measures
Kolmogorov-Smirnov (2)	Ordinal, interval, or ratio data not meeting t test assumptions and not grouped as cumulative frequencies, independent measures
Wilcoxon signed-rank (2)	Ordinal, interval, or ratio data not meeting t test assumptions, paired measures
Kruskall-Wallis (3)	Ordinal, interval, or ratio data not meeting ANOVA assumptions, independent measures
Friedman (3)	Ordinal, interval, or ratio data not meeting ANOVA assumptions, paired measures

5)   one-sided versus two-sided significance tests

Another criterion used for selection of the proper statistical test is whether the test should be one-sided or two-sided. Two-sided or two-tailed significance tests examine the probability that the investigational drug would be superior or inferior to the control drug. A one-sided or one-tailed test assumes that a difference occurs in one direction, usually that the investigational drug is superior to the drug used in the control group. One-sided tests are more powerful than two-sided tests because the focus on one direction reduces the variability of the data. Despite the value of using a one-sided test, there are numerous limitations which minimize its use (Table 17-18). Two-sided tests are usually preferred because there is a lower likelihood of biased interpretation by the trial investigators. Use of one-sided tests of significance should always be clearly noted by the investigators.[6,20,23,45,47,57-62]

Table 17-18.   Limitations of Using One-sided Significance Tests

Limitation	Description
Lack of uniformity	Arbitrary use of one-sided or two-sided tests creates an inconsistency in the reporting of p values
Lack of theoretical support	Prior research or theory rarely enables the investigator to confidently predict that the investigational drug will only have a positive effect
Exaggeration of differences	One-sided tests tend to exaggerate the importance of marginal therapeutic differences

6)   reporting the statistical analysis

Ideally, investigators should refrain from simply stating what test of significance was used during the statistical analysis. Statements such as "we used t tests, Chi square, and Fisher's exact test" are acceptable only if supplemented with a clear description of the statistical analysis plan in which the tests are used. Although often limited by journal space restrictions, investigators should discuss their assumptions about the data and the expectations regarding the direction in which the effect will occur.[5,63]

d.   Planned statistical analysis

Planned statistical analysis involves the development of hypotheses or objectives before the research and implementation of a structured analysis plan to test the hypotheses in an efficient manner. Unplanned statistical analysis is less structured and more likely to identify chance differences between the experimental and control groups. The value of a planned statistical analysis is illustrated in the analysis of multiple responses or endpoints. Reported results of many clinical drug trials often include analysis of different aspects of the patient's response to the drug treatment. However, the use of significance tests to compare the experimental and control groups on each response could increase the likelihood that a significant difference will be detected by chance (Type I error or alpha error). A tendency also exists to concentrate on those responses which are most favorable to the investigator's hypotheses, even if the particular result has a low theoretical plausibility or lacks prior data to support it. To offset the possibility of emphasizing false results, investigators should clearly designate at the beginning of the clinical drug trial the endpoints or responses which will be the main criteria for assessing drug treatment differences.[2,4,6,18,20,37,49,64,65]

A major source of unplanned statistical analysis is the evaluation of particular categories or subgroups of patients (e.g., women, aged patients, certain symptoms of the disease state, racial minorities) to determine whether they will respond differently to the investigational drug. Subgroup analysis is done primarily to assess interactions within the data which occur when the reported drug effects differ among various subgroups. An example of an interaction effect would be a report that an investigational drug is more effective and safe in patients suffering from osteoarthritis of the knee compared to patients suffering from osteoarthritis of the elbow.[20,66]

Conclusions based on subgroup analysis can be misleading. Most clinical drug trials do not have enough patients enrolled to fulfill the requirements for appropriate statistical testing of subgroup effects. In addition, the large number of possible subgroups that can be analyzed creates an opportunity to identify only those subgroups most responsive to the investigational drug, especially if the analysis is done in an unplanned manner. Some suggested guidelines to use for assessing differences in subgroups are listed in Table 17-19.[19,20,64,66]

Table 17-19.   Suggested Guidelines for Subgroup Analysis[19,66]

Guideline	Description
Number of tested hypotheses	Only a small number of hypotheses should be tested to reduce the likelihood for chance detection of subgroup differences
Type of hypotheses tested	*Post hoc* hypotheses should be tested sparingly because they are more prone to identify false results than are *a priori* hypotheses
Statistical significance	The statistical tests should show subgroup differences significant at least at the $p<0.05$ level, although a level of $p<0.01$ is preferred
Size of group difference	The subgroup difference should be of sufficient size to be considered clinically important
Consistency from prior search	The subgroup difference is considered to be more plausible if it is consistent with results of prior research
Presence of indirect evidence	Theoretical or biological evidence should exist to support the credibility of the subgroup difference

19. Were the results of the significance testing interpreted correctly?

Many of the problems associated with misinterpreting the results of significance testing involve a misunderstanding of the p value. From a statistical standpoint, significance tests provide the probability of making a Type I or alpha error, which is the likelihood that an observed difference is due to a chance occurrence. The probability is represented by the p value, which is designed to help the investigator guard against surprise or unexpected findings. In order to improve the understanding of the p value, an attempt has been made to standardize certain interpretations (Table 17-20). According to guidelines indicated in Table 17-20, statistical significance occurs with any p value less than 0.05, which generally means that the investigator is 95% confident that the differences observed are not due to chance. The choice of $p < 0.05$ as statistically significant is an arbitrary cutoff that was originally developed for use in quality control studies where the emphasis was on making decisions for improving the manufacturing process. Thus, a p value such as $p < 0.055$ is not considered statistically significant because it is rounded to $p < 0.06$ while $p < 0.054$ is considered statistically significant because it can be rounded to $p < 0.05$.[6,18,19,37,47,63,67]

Table 17-20.   Standard Interpretation of p Values[37,47]

p Value	Interpretation
p=0.06 and greater	Not statistically significant
0.05> p >0.01	Statistically significant[a]
0.01> p >0.001	Very statistically significant[b]
p <0.001	Highly statistically significant[b]

[a]   The value is more commonly stated as p < 0.05. Thus, any value of p equal to 0.05 or less is considered statistically significant.

[b]   The two interpretations are sometimes combined so that any value of p equal to 0.01 or less is considered highly statistically significant.

Despite attempts to standardize interpretation of p values as indicated in Table 17-20, p values are often misinterpreted in the reporting of results of a clinical drug trial. Investigators sometimes place undue importance on a p value of 0.05 or less by implying that such a result, based on statistical significance alone, is clinically important. Statistical significance does not provide much information about the magnitude or importance of the observed difference (see Chapter 18, Question 22). Rather, statistical significance indicates that a strong probability exists that a nonchance difference between the experimental and control groups was observed. The proper interpretation of statistically nonsignificant results is that a strong likelihood exists that no differences were observed between the experimental and control groups. Investigators should refrain from merely stating that a result is "statistically significant" without stating the test statistic used and the observed p value. In addition, misleading statements such as "almost significant" or "there is a trend toward significance" for p values greater than 0.05 should be avoided. For studies in which no differences were found, discussion of the probability of making a Type II or beta error should be included (see Question 20).[6,18,19,37,47,63,67]

P values are based on mathematical models or probability estimations. The correctness of those values depends on the extent to which the underlying assumptions are met by the data collected. For parametric tests such as the t test or analysis of variance, these assumptions include normally distributed and continuously scaled data, independent measures, and equal variability among the trial groups (Table 17-15). Significance tests do not address possible problems with the trial design, especially those problems which may result in trial groups that are not directly comparable. Any assessment of significance tests should include a review of the steps that the investigators undertook to ensure group comparability. Such steps include random assignment of patients, proper management of data collection, maintenance of similar patient dropout rates in each group, and analysis of possible group differences. P values are also affected by the number of the patients in the clinical drug trial. Trials with large numbers of patients are more likely to result in statistically significant differences than trials with small numbers (see Question 20). Causal relationships are difficult to establish solely through the use of statistical tests (see Chapter 18, Question 21).[1,23,25,47,51,52,63]

20. *What influence does the number of patients analyzed have on the interpretation of the reported results?*

Statistical interpretation of the differences between the experimental and control groups is strongly influenced by the number of patients enrolled. An assessment of that influence can be made through the estimation of the power of a statistical test. Power is defined as the probability that the statistical test will detect true differences between the experimental and control groups (Type II or beta error) and is calculated by subtracting the Type II error probability from 1. The power of a statistical test depends of several factors: the size of the sample, the desired size of the difference to be detected, the amount of variation in the data collected, or the desired alpha level for making a Type I error (Table 17-21). There are a number of formulas available to calculate the power of a statistical test and the calculations are usually done before the trial is implemented. However, power calculations should also be done after the trial data are collected when more precise information needed for the calculation is usually available.[6,46,68-73]

Table 17-21.   Factors Influencing the Power of a Statistical Text

Factor	Influence on Power
Sample size	Increases with the sample size
Size of difference	Increases as the expected size of the difference to be detected between the experimental and control groups increases
Variability	Increases as the variability among the data decreases
Type I (alpha) error	Increases as the probability of making a Type I error increases

Unlike Type I or alpha errors, there is no traditional consensus about the acceptable level of power of a statistical test. The Type II error rate is often set at a maximum value of 20% which sets the minimum acceptable power level at 80% (power = 1 - Type II error rate). The acceptance of setting the power level at 80% illustrates the greater emphasis that investigators put on avoiding Type I errors (with an acceptable level of five percent) than Type II errors. Reliance on a less conservative power level can result in investigators missing clinically important differences between the experimental and control group or clinically important but relatively rare drug side effects.[25,38,71,74,75]

The primary way in which investigators avoid the effects of low statistical power is to enroll an adequate number of patients in the trial. Although the actual number of patients enrolled in a clinical drug trial is often influenced more by factors such as patient availability, cost constraints, trial duration, or government regulations, estimation of the desired number should be based on statistical theory. The statistical estimation is based on the variability of the data collected and the anticipated size of the differences to be detected. An example of the estimation is illustrated by the hypothetical example shown in Table 17-22 in which the effectiveness of a new antiarrhythmic drug in reducing the incidence of atrial fibrillation (AF) is compared to standard treatment. In this example, the incidence of atrial fibrillation remains constant at 50% for the control group. The table indicates that a larger number of patients are needed as the expected difference between the experimental and control group becomes smaller. In addition, increasing the power of the test requires increasing the number of patients enrolled in the clinical drug trial.[23,38,69,72]

Table 17-22.   Estimated Number of Patients Needed for the Control and Experimental Groups in a Clinical Trial of a New Antiarrhythmic Drug

Incidence of AF[a]			Number of Patients Needed in Each Group[b]		
EXP	CTL	DIFF	N_{10}[c]	N_{20}[d]	N_{50}[e]
5	50	45	23	19	12
10	50	40	30	24	15
20	50	30	58	45	26
30	50	20	134	103	56
40	50	10	538	407	210
45	50	5	2130	1600	806

[a]   Represents the percentage of patients in the sample with atrial fibrillation (AF). The percentage was held constant at 50% for patients in the control group.

[b]   The number of patients needed is calculated from the formulas recommended by Borenstein and Cohen.[76] The Chi Square statistic (with the Yates correction) is used to assess statistical significance. Power=1-beta (probability of Type II error). The p value is assumed to be equal to 0.05.

[c] N_{10} is the power level of 0.90 and represents a 10% probability that a Type II error could occur.

[d] N_{20} is the power level of 0.80 and represents a 20% probability that a Type II error could occur. It is the most commonly used level.

[e] N_{50} is the power level of 0.50 and represents a 50% probability that a Type II error could occur.

AF=Atrial Fibrillation EXP=Experimental group CTL=Control group
DIFF=Expected percentage difference between experimental and control group

Clinical drug trials with low power are likely to report no differences between the experimental and control group, even when actual differences exists. These results could impede future research on the investigational drug or misrepresent the actual differences between the drug and standard drug treatment. It is also possible that a large number of clinical drug trials could report conflicting results primarily because of the different number of subjects used in each trial.[19,20,71,72,77]

References

1.   Koch GG, Sollecito WA. Statistical considerations in the design, analysis and interpretation of comparative clinical studies. *Drug Info J* 1984;18:131-51.
2.   Bailar JC. Science, statistics, and deception. *Ann Intern Med* 1986;104:259-60.

3. Pocock SJ. Basic principles of statistical analysis. In Pocock SJ, ed. Clinical trials: a practical approach. New York: J Wiley and Sons, 1983:188-209.
4. Walker AM. Reporting the results of epidemiologic studies. *Am J Pub Health* 1986;76:556-8.
5. Moses LE. Statistical concepts fundamental to investigations. In Bailar JC and Mosteller F, eds. Medical use of statistics. Boston: NEJM books, 1992:5-25.
6. Elenbaas RM, Elenbaas JK, Cuddy PG. Evaluating the medical literature, part II: statistical analysis. *Ann Emerg Med* 1983;12:610-20.
7. Pocock SJ. Protocol deviations. In Pocock SJ, ed. Clinical Trials: a practical approach. New York: J Wiley and Sons, 1983:176-186.
8. Kramer MS, Shapiro SH. Scientific challenges in the application of randomized trials. *JAMA* 1984;252:2739-45.
9. Freedman LS. The effect of partial noncompliance on the power of a clinical trial. *Controlled Clinical Trials* 1990;11:157-68.
10. Polk RE, Hepler CD. Controversies in antimicrobial therapy: critical analysis of clinical trials. *Am J Hosp Pharm* 1986;43:630-40.
11. Moscucci M, Byrne L, Weintraub M, Cox C. Blinding, unblinding, and the placebo effect: an analysis of patients' guesses of treatment assignment in a double-blind clinical trial. *Clin Pharmacol Ther* 1987;41:259-65.
12. Pocock SJ. Clinical trials: a practical approach. New York: Wiley & Sons, 1983:111.
13. Hallstrom A, Davis K. Imbalance in treatment assignments in stratified blocked randomization. *Controlled Clin Trials* 1988;9:375-82.
14. Bailar JC, Mosteller F. Guidelines for statistical reporting in articles for medical journals. In Bailar JC and Mosteller F, eds. Medical use of statistics. Boston: NEJM books, 1992:313-331.
15. United States Pharmacopeia. Drug information for the health professional. 13th edition. Rockville. United States Pharmacopeial Convention, Inc., 1993
16. Hamilton CW. How to write and publish scientific papers: scribing information for pharmacists. *Am J Hosp Pharm* 1992;49:2477-84.
17. Kirwin JR. Clinical trials: why not do them properly? *Ann Rheum Dis* 1982;41:551-52.
18. Barnes RW. Understanding investigative clinical trials. *J Vasc Surg* 1989;9:609-18.
19. Pocock SJ, Hughes MD. Estimation issues in clinical trials and overviews. *Stat Med* 1990;9:657-71.
20. Pocock SJ. Current issues in the design and interpretation of clinical trials. *Br Med J* 1985;290:39-42.
21. Lavori PW, Louis TA, Bailar JC, Polansky M. Designs for experiments-parallel comparisons of treatment. *N Engl J Med* 1983;309:1291-8.
22. Pocock SJ. Further aspects of data analysis. In Pocock SJ, ed. Clinical trials: a practical approach. New York: J Wiley and Sons, 1983: 211-233.
23. Bolton S. Pharmaceutical statistics. 2nd ed. New York: Marcel Dekker, 1990.
24. Sackett DL. How to read clinical journal: I. Why to read them and how to start reading them critically. *CMA Journal* 1981;124:555-8.
25. Kirk RE. Experimental design. 2nd ed. Pacific Grove, Ca: Brooks/Cole, 1982.
26. O'Brien PC, Shampo MA. Statistics for clinicians: introduction. *Mayo Clin Proc* 1981;56:45-6.

27. Feinstein AR. Clinical biostatistics IV: statistical "malpractice"--and the responsibility of a consultant. *Clin Pharmacol Ther* 1970;11:898-914.

28. Gaddis ML, Gaddis GM. Introduction to biostatistics: part 1, basic concepts. *Ann Emerg Med* 1990;19:86-89.

29. Gehlbach SH. Interpreting the medical literature: a clinician's guide: practical epidemiology for clinicians. 2nd ed. New York: Macmillan Publishing Company, 1988:70-74.

30. Riegelman RK, Hirsch RP. Studying a study and testing a test: how to read the medical literature. 2nd ed. Boston: Little Brown, 1989.

31. Norman GR, Streiner DL. PDQ statistics. Philadelphia: BC Decker, 1986.

32. Gaddis GM, Gaddis ML. Introduction to biostatistics: part 2, descriptive statistics. *Ann Emerg Med* 1990;19:309-15.

33. Matthews DE, Farwell VT. Using and understanding medical statistics. 2nd ed. Switzerland: Karger, 1988.

34. O'Brien PC, Shampo MA. Statistics for clinicians: 1. Descriptive statistics. *Mayo Clin Proc* 1981;56:47-9.

35. O'Brien PC, Shampo MA. Statistics for clinicians: 2. Graphic displays-histograms, frequency polygons, and cumulative distribution polygons. *Mayo Clin Proc* 1981;56:126-8.

36. O'Brien PC, Shampo MA. Statistics for clinicians: 3. Graphic displays-scatter diagrams. *Mayo Clin Proc* 1981;56:196-7.

37. Bennett RW, Popovich NG. Statistical inference as applied to bioavailability data--a guide for the practicing pharmacists. *Am J Hosp Pharm* 1977;34:712-23.

38. Campbell MJ, Machin D. Medical statistics: a commonsense approach. New York: J Wiley and Sons, 1990.

39. Gaddis ML, Gaddis GM. Introduction to biostatistics: part 6, correlation and regression. *Ann Emerg Med* 1990;19:1462-3.

40. Liebetrau AM. Measures of association. Newbury Park, Ca.: Sage Publications, 1983.

41. O'Brien PC, Shampo MA. Statistics for clinicians: 7. Regression. *Mayo Clin Proc* 1981;56:452-4.

42. Mosteller F. Writing about numbers. In Bailar JC and Mosteller F, eds. Medical use of statistics. Boston: NEJM books, 1992: 375-89.

43. Ehrenberg ASC. The problem of numeracy. *Am Stat* 1981;35:67-71.

44. Zelterman D, Louis TA. Contingency tables in medical studies. In Bailar JC and Mosteller F, eds. Medical use of statistics. Boston: NEJM books, 1992: 293-311.

45. Elenbaas JK, Cuddy PG, Elenbaas RM. Evaluating the medical literature part III: results and discussion. *Ann Emerg Med* 1983;12:679-686.

46. Gaddis GM, Gaddis ML. Introduction to biostatistics: part 3, sensitivity, specificity, predictive value and hypothesis testing. *Ann Emerg Med* 1990;19:591-7.

47. Ware JH, Mosteller F, Delgaudo F, Donnelly C, Ingelfinger JA. P Values. In Bailar JC and Mosteller F, eds. Medical use of statistics. Boston: NEJM books 1992:181-200.

48. Gaddis GM, Gaddis ML. Introduction to biostatistics: part 4, statistical inference techniques in hypothesis testing. *Ann Emerg Med* 1990;19:820-5.

49. Saville DJ. Multiple comparison procedures: the practical solution. *Am Stat* 1990;44:174-180.

50. O'Brien PC, Shampo MA. Statistics for clinicians: 8. Comparing two proportions: the relative deviate test and Chi square equivalent. *Mayo Clin Proc* 1981;56:513-5.

51. O'Brien PC, Shampo MA. Statistics for clinicians: 5. One sample of paired observations (paired t test). *Mayo Clin Proc* 1981;56:324-6.

52. Boyce EG, Nappi JM. Is there significance beyond the t-test? *Drug Intell Clin Pharm* 1988;22:334-5.

53. Pathek D. Parametric vs nonparametric statistics: a dilemma for the clinical researcher. *Drug Intell Clin Pharm* 1979;13:441-2.

54. Gaddis GM, Gaddis ML. Introduction to biostatistics: part 5, statistical inference techniques in hypothesis testing with nonparametric data. *Ann Emerg Med* 1990;19:1054-9.

55. Godfrey K. Comparing the means of several groups. *N Engl J Med* 1985;313:1450-6.

56. Iverson GR, Norpoth H. Analysis of variance. Newbury Park, Ca.: Sage Publications, 1987.

57. Salsburg D. Use of restricted significance tests in clinical trials: beyond the one vs two-tailed controversy. *Controlled Clinical Trials* 1989;10:71-82.

58. Boissel JP. Some thoughts on two-tailed tests (and two-sided designs). *Controlled Clinical Trials* 1988;9:385-6.

59. Peace KE. Some thoughts on one-tailed tests. *Controlled Clinical Trials* 1988;9:383-4.

60. Fleiss JL. One-tailed versus two-tailed tests: rebuttal. *Controlled Clinical Trials* 1988;10:227-30.

61. Goodman S. One-sided or two-sided p values? *Controlled Clinical Trials* 1988;9:387-8.

62. Mckinney WP, Young MJ, Hartz A, Lee MB. The inexact use of Fisher's exact test in six major medical journals. *JAMA* 1989;261:3430-3.

63. Henzel RE. Tests of significance. Newbury Park, Ca.: Sage Publications, 1976.

64. Thompson DW. Statistical criteria in the interpretation of epidemiologic data. *Am J Pub Health* 1987;77:191-4.

65. Tukey JW. Some thoughts on clinical trials, especially problems of multiplicity. *Science* 1977;198:679-84.

66. Oxman AD, Guyatt GH. A consumer's guide to subgroup analysis. *Ann Intern Med* 1992;116:76-84.

67. Fleiss JL. Significance tests have a role in epidemologic research: reaction. *Am J Pub Health* 1987;76:559-60.

68. Kupper LL, Hafner KB. How appropriate are popular sample size formulas? *Am Stat* 1989;43:101-5.

69. Cohen J. Statistical power analysis for the behavioral sciences. 2nd ed. Hillsdale, NJ: L Erlbaum Associates, 1988.

70. Moussa MAA. Exact conditional, and predictive power in planning clinical trials. *Controlled Clinical Trials* 1989;10:376-85.

71. Altman DG. Size of clinical trials. *Br Med J* 1983;286:1842-3.

72. Mosteller F, Gilbert JP, McPeek B. Reporting standards and research strategies for controlled trials: agenda for the editor. *Controlled Clinical Trials* 1980;1:37-58.

73. Browner WS, Newman TB. Are all significant P values created equal? *N Engl J Med* 1987;257:2459-63.

74. Schneiweiss F, Uthoff VA. Sample size and postmarketing surveillance. *Drug Info J* 1985;19:13-6.

75. Freiman JA, Chalmers TC, Smith H, Kuebler RR. The importance of beta, the Type II error and sample size in the design and interpretation of the randomize control trial. *N Engl J Med* 1978;299:690-4.

76. Borenstein M, Cohen J. Statistical power analysis: a computer program. Hillsdale, NJ: L Erlbaum Associates, 1988.
77. Arkin CF, Wachtel MS. How many patients are necessary to assess test performance? *JAMA* 1990;263:275-78.

Checklist Questions

21. *Was a causal relationship firmly established between the results reported and the use of the investigational drug?*

22. *How clinically important are the reported differences between the experimental and control groups?*

23. *Have the investigators established that the reported results can be extrapolated to everyday clinical practice?*

Discussion

The final part of an article describing a clinical drug trial usually involves a discussion of the reported results and a conclusion regarding the implications of the trial findings. Publishers of journals vary in their policies regarding how the final section is organized: some require that the discussion and conclusion sections be separated while others suggest that the sections be combined. Unfortunately, a lengthy and comprehensive discussion section would be unusual in most publications because of space limitations. Thus, the investigators are often limited in the extent to which they can discuss the reported results of the clinical drug trial.

The discussion and conclusion section should focus on providing the investigators' interpretation of the trial results. This interpretation includes a discussion about how the results answer the research questions described in the trial objectives or research hypotheses, their importance to everyday clinical practice, and their implications for future research. New and important results should be emphasized and linked with previous research or with current knowledge. Recommendations regarding follow-up research to confirm the results can be provided, especially if contradictions are reported. The investigators should explain the implications of reported results that contradict other research on the same drug treatment. Results inconsistent with previous hypotheses can lead to new scientific insight. However, inconsistent results can also be due to poor research design, differences in the trial design or patient population used, or an excessively biased interpretation by the investigators. Although the applicability of the results to everyday clinical practice should be discussed, overly enthusiastic extrapolation should be avoided. Most importantly, investigators need to clearly state their conclusions along with supporting evidence from the trial results.[1-3]

Explanation of Checklist Questions

21. Was a causal relationship firmly established between the results reported and the use of the investigational drug?

The primary purpose of the discussion and conclusion sections is for the investigators to establish whether the investigational drug was effective and safe. While no consistent procedure is routinely followed to establish efficacy and safety, the discussion should include a definition of the causal relationship between the investigational drug and the observed clinical outcomes. In addition, a description of the method used to assess the relationship and to eliminate other potential causative factors should be included.

The definition of causality is based on the science of philosophy and refers to a specific set (or locus) of events that take place during a specified time frame (past, present, or future). The definition of a causal relationship for the efficacy of an anti-arrhythmic drug, for example, could be the elimination of preventricular contractions in patients within one month of first taking the investigational drug. Causality is determined either retrospectively or prospectively. The retrospective approach would be the identification of an effect that has already occurred followed by an assessment of its possible causes. The prospective method would involve a prediction that a significant number of patients exposed to the investigational drug will respond in a pre-determined manner. Case control studies are often designed to address retrospective causal propositions while cohort studies or clinical drug trials are most effective for developing prospective causal explanations.[4-7]

A typical causal proposition in a clinical drug trial would be the suggestion that the investigational drug caused an observed improvement in the clinical condition of the patient compared to patients receiving placebo or a standard drug treatment. The implication would be that the investigational drug altered the natural course of the disease, resulting in improved clinical outcomes. Another causal proposition may be that factors other than the investigational drug caused some or all of the adverse drug reactions reported in the trial. These propositions should be evaluated directly or indirectly through the use of widely accepted criteria for assessing causality (Table 18-1). Because most of the criteria are not systematically addressed by investigators in the discussion or conclusion sections, the health care practitioner needs to read the sections carefully to determine whether sufficient evidence is provided for a causal relationship to be established. Meeting all of the criteria described in Table 18-1 would not unequivocally establish that the investigational drug caused the clinical outcomes, particularly if the design of the trial has flaws such as nonrandom assignment of patients, lack of double blind techniques, or poor measures. Nevertheless, the probability of a causal relationship existing between the investigational drug and the clinical outcomes increases as the number of criteria met increases.[8-11]

Table 18-1. Criteria for Establishing Causality in Clinical Drug Trials[8-11]

Criteria	Description
Temporal relationship	The clinical outcome should clearly occur after (not before) the investigational drug is administered to the patient
Strength	The incidence of the clinical outcome reported in the experimental group should be higher than the incidence reported in the control group
Consistency	The clinical outcomes reported in the clinical drug trial have been reported in other trials with the same investigational drug or with other drugs within the same class
Clinical plausibility	The relationship is clinically probable based on the current understanding of the investigational drug and the disease under treatment
Specificity	The clinical outcome has a high probability of occurring when the investigational drug is given and is likely to be absent when the drug is not present
Dose-response effect	The severity or size of the clinical outcome increases with increasing doses or duration of the investigational drug
Ruling out confounding factors	The effects of other plausible alternate explanations (e.g., other drugs taken concurrently, the presence of other medical conditions) are eliminated as possible explanations for the clinical outcome

a.   Temporal relationship

The primary objective in establishing a temporal relationship is to ensure that the observed clinical outcomes occurred after (not before) the investigational drug was administered. This objective is often difficult to establish because the clinical outcomes may be due to many factors, especially the natural course of the disease. Theoretically, a randomized controlled trial (RCT) should be effective in establishing a temporal relationship through the use of control groups containing similar patients (see Chapter 15). Because case control or cohort studies do not routinely possess similar characteristics as a randomized control trial, a temporal relationship is more difficult to establish (see Chapter 12). Establishment of a temporal relationship in a randomized control trial is not guaranteed. Protocol deviations such as treating patients with a diagnosis lacking the expected outcome, patient noncompliance, concurrent use of interacting drugs, and variations in the data collection procedures can make establishing the temporal relationship more difficult (see Chapter 17, Question 14).[7,8,10]

b. Strength

The strength of a causal relationship is determined by the relative frequency of the expected clinical outcome in the experimental group compared to the control group. The strength is sometimes expressed as the relative risk, which is defined by the following formula:

$$\text{relative risk} = \frac{\text{incidence of clinical outcome in experimental group}}{\text{incidence of clinical outcome in control group}}$$

There are no consistent guidelines that indicate the appropriate size of the relative risk needed to suggest a causal relationship. Nevertheless, a relative risk ratio of 10 (meaning that the clinical outcome is 10 times more likely to occur in the experimental group than the control group) would be better than a relative risk ratio of 2. However, relative risk ratios are sometimes misleading if the incidence of the effect is comparatively rare, such as with many adverse drug reactions. A relative risk ratio of three may appear important but it may only indicate that the effect is likely to occur just three times in an experimental group of 1000 patients compared to once in a control group of similar size. Like temporal relationships, the strength of a causal relationship is established most easily in randomized controlled trials (see Chapter 15). Non-randomized clinical drug trials are less likely to accurately estimate the strength of the relationship because there is less information available about the similarity of the experimental and control patients. Even randomization does not ensure accurate estimation of the causal relationship's strength. Differences between the experimental and control group could be distorted in clinical drug trials that contain a small number of patients.[8-10,12-14]

c. Consistency

Consistency is based on the expected reproducibility of the causal relationship. While reproducibility of the relationship can sometimes occur in the same trial if patients are re-exposed to the investigational drug, the usual method to establish consistency is through the examination of previous research by the investigators. The examination should include references to similar trials of the investigational drug. Inconsistent trial results reported by the investigators should be justified in order to ensure that the results are not due to poor research design or biased interpretation of the data. Information about drugs from the same class is often used to establish consistency because of the paucity of information that is usually available about an investigational drug.[1,2,8,10]

d. Clinical plausibility

Clinical plausibility refers to the existing prior evidence supporting the causal relationship. Assessing the clinical plausibility of the causal relationship is similar to establishing the relationship's consistency. The investigators need to provide background information from prior research and existing clinical practice about the expected and unexpected effects of the investigational drug. Because almost any potential causal relationship can be made to sound clinically plausible, the investigators need to provide sufficient background information to justify their assertions. Information from drugs of the same class may need to be used in situations where the newness of the investigational drug restricts the availability of similar information.[1,2,8,10,15]

e. Specificity

Specificity is determined by the distinctness of the causal relationship. The expected clinical outcome should appear after the investigational drug is administered but not if the drug was not present. Specificity is difficult to establish in a clinical drug trial because most clinical outcomes have multiple causes besides the investigational drug. In addition, investigational drugs rarely cause the expected clinical outcomes in all patients. Specificity may be better assessed in trials in which selected subgroups of patients are present which uniformly respond to the investigational drug or in trials in which the expected clinical outcome is clearly established prior to the trial.[8,10,16,17]

f. Dose-response effect

The dose-response effect consists of an expected change in the clinical outcomes when the dose or duration of the investigational drug is changed. The relationship should be predetermined based on prior evidence and usually consists of measuring the clinical outcomes after various dosages of the investigational drug are administered. Because of the methodological and analytical complexities of a clinical drug trial involving different doses of the investigational drug, the dose-response relationship is infrequently assessed in a single trial. Nevertheless, the clinical outcome of a trial using a fixed dose of the investigational drug can be compared with prior research or existing clinical practice where different doses of the drug are administered. A dose-response effect would be difficult to assess in those conditions in which a quantitative assessment of the patient response is not possible. An example may be the evaluation of an anti-infective drug in which the clinical outcome is measured by the nominal scale of presence or absence of symptoms. No range of response would be possible with this type of scale (see Chapter 17, Question 16).[8,10]

g. Ruling out confounding factors

Of all the criteria discussed in Table 18-1, the ruling out of confounding factors is probably the most important. The process involves identifying possible alternative reasons for the clinical outcomes observed, and assessing the probability that the alternate reasons influenced the result. Like the other criteria, using a design that includes the features of a randomized controlled trial with an adequate number of patients would be the most effective strategy for ruling out confounding factors. In addition, stratification of the patients by possible confounding factors (such as age or gender) prior to assignment to the experimental or control groups may be effective. Statistical analysis may be used to assess the possible effects of confounding factors in those clinical drug trials lacking the features of a randomized controlled trial, using a small number of patients, or lacking stratification. Though not as effective as manipulation of the trial design, statistical analysis is useful if it compares the drug effects by subgroups of patients or statistically tests for the probability of alternate hypotheses. Regardless of the approach used, the investigators should clearly provide evidence to support their assumption that alternative explanations besides the investigational drug were less likely to influence the reported results.[5,7,11,18-21]

22. *How clinically important are the reported differences between the experimental and control groups?*

The importance of an observed difference between the experimental and control groups cannot be clearly assessed unless the likelihood that the difference is due to chance (statistical significance) is known. The larger the trial, the lower the probability that a chance difference occurred (see Chapter 17, Question 19). However, differences that are statistically significant may not be clinically important. Statistical significance is determined quantitatively using precise guidelines. Clinical significance is more subjective and is dependent on the opinion of the health care practitioner and patient. While judgment of statistical significance is based on a probability assessment of the results reported, clinical significance is based on previously reported knowledge (Table 18-2). Results that are statistically important but are not supported by previous knowledge should be interpreted cautiously. Statistically significant differences are sometimes erroneously accepted as being clinically important despite the presence of severe limitations in the trial methodology or in the analysis of the results.[22-27]

Table 18-2.   Comparison of Statistical and Clinical Significance[28]

Characteristic	Statistical Significance	Clinical Significance
Purpose	Detect nonchance differences	Assess importance of difference
Criteria	$p < 0.05$	Expert/personal opinion
Determinants	Sample size Patient variability Accurate/reliable measures	Extent of change in clinical practice or change in quality of life measures (e.g., improved patient comfort, mortality)

a. Use of confidence intervals (CIs)

Significance tests only determine whether the results are statistically significant and provide limited information about the magnitude or importance of the difference between the experimental and control group. Confidence intervals are often recommended as an alternative method to significance tests because they provide a range in which the actual difference is likely to exist (see Chapter 17, Question 16). Like significance tests, the degree of confidence that the actual value is within the reported range of values is traditionally set at 95%. An example of using the confidence interval would be reporting that an investigational anti-hypertensive drug reduced diastolic blood pressure by 20% compared to controls. The investigators may report that the results were statistically significant (p< 0.05). The results would be more informative, however, if the confidence interval of the difference was also reported. A description of the confidence interval being between 3% to 40% mmHg indicates that a 95% chance exists that the actual difference is between the two numbers reported. A narrower confidence interval provides a better estimate of the actual value compared to larger intervals. A confidence interval that includes 1 (such as 0.7% to 30%) indicates that there is a strong probability that no difference exists between the experimental and control groups.[23,29,30-33]

The past misuse of significance tests has generated numerous recommendations that the tests be replaced by confidence intervals, particularly in case control or cohort studies. Although overdependence on significance tests leads to incomplete information, p values provide details that are typically not present when only confidence intervals are reported. The statement that p=0.0001 gives a clear indication of the likelihood that the observed difference is not due to chance. In addition, significance tests are based on pre-specified criteria that require clear-cut and explicit decisions about the data collected. Thus, it may be preferable to cite both significance tests and confidence intervals when reporting the results of the clinical drug trial.[2,18,23,31-38]

Effective use of both the p value and the confidence interval was demonstrated in the reported results of a clinical drug trial evaluating the effectiveness and safety of sumatriptan for the treatment of migraine headache.[39]

> "As compared with the placebo group at 60 minutes (after treatment), 47% more patients (95% confidence interval, 38% to 57%) who had received 6 mg of sumatriptan and 54% more patients (95% confidence interval, 43% to 65%) who had received 8 mg of sumatriptan had improvements in the severity of headache (p<0.001 for both comparisons). A complete resolution of pain also occurred in a significantly higher proportion of patients treated with either dose of sumatriptan than of patients given placebo (p<0.001)."

23. Have the investigators established that the reported results can be extrapolated to everyday clinical practice?

After the results of the clinical drug trial are reported, the investigators need to assess how they can be applied to patients in everyday clinical practice. This assessment focuses on the external validity or applicability of the reported results and is sometimes referred to as extrapolation, estimation, or induction. Extrapolation of the reported results is probably the most difficult task in scientific literature evaluation and involves making inferences beyond the results of the clinical drug trial. The inferences are often needed because of the constraints placed on the trial design to insure that the trial followed the appropriate scientific guidelines. Despite the difficulty associated with assessing the applicability of the reported results, extrapolation is necessary if the investigational drug is going to be used properly. Unwillingness to extrapolate limits the research results to a narrow range of patients similar to those in the trial and unnecessarily restricts the potential value of the investigational drug.[11,16,24,40,41]

Assessing the applicability of the trial results usually involves comparing the characteristics of the trial with similar characteristics that are likely to be present in everyday clinical practice. Some of the characteristics are related to the patient (age, gender, race, or medical condition), medical setting, or the drug regimen used (see Chapter 14, Question 6). Other characteristics are related to the methodology used, such as the potential biases in the subject selection procedure (see Chapter 14, Question 7) or poor measures used for assessing the efficacy and safety of the clinical drug trial (see Chapter 16, Questions 12-13). Regardless of the characteristics assessed, the extrapolation process is full of potential errors (Table 18-3). Even if few errors are made in extrapolation, health care practitioners should be cautious about changing their behavior based on the results of a single trial. Results need to be repeated and experience gained in broader populations before the true efficacy and safety of the investigational drug is established.[17,26,42-44]

Table 18-3.   Common Errors of Extrapolation[40,45]

Errors of Extrapolation	Description
Design biases	Ignoring potential subject selection bias, biased measurement of results, presence of confounding factors
Wrong hypotheses	Developing hypotheses or conclusions based on unplanned analysis of the data
Selective emphasis of subgroup differences	Choosing to emphasize only results that support trial hypotheses
Wrong statistical methods	Using descriptive statistics to emphasize certain inferences and choosing the wrong significance test
Selective reporting	Emphasizing only certain aspects of the trial results

a.   Design biases

A major error of extrapolation occurs when investigators ignore the limitations of the trial design, particularly the potential differences between the sample of patients and those who will use the drug in clinical practice. Poor extrapolation will occur when the differences between these two groups of patients are not adequately evaluated. Because most patients in clinical drug trials are not selected randomly from the general population, attention needs to focus on what biases are involved in the selection process and the effect of the biases on the extrapolation of the results (see Chapter 14). Another potential limitation of the trial design is the biased measurement of the efficacy and safety of the investigational drug. It is possible that the drug effects were measured for an insufficient length of time or without blinded observers. In addition, the wrong type of measures may have been used (see Chapter 16). Poor extrapolation also occurs when possible confounding factors or alternate explanations are inappropriately ignored (see Question 21).

b. Wrong hypotheses

Hypotheses are developed prior to the trial (*a priori* hypothesis) or after the data are collected (*post hoc* or *post priori* hypotheses). Poor extrapolation of the results is more likely to occur if the experiment is based on *post priori* hypotheses rather than *a priori* hypotheses because the former are more likely to be affected by the data collected in the trial than by the existing knowledge or theories about the investigational drug. While useful for suggesting the direction of future research efforts, *post priori* hypotheses should be avoided or used carefully when the reported results are extrapolated to the clinical practice setting (see Chapter 17, Question 18).

c. Selective emphasis of subgroup differences

Analyzing subgroups of patients is appropriate to determine if more specific differences may occur between the experimental and control group. However, unplanned subgroup analysis is prone to a number of errors such as testing an excessive number of subgroup differences, choosing the wrong statistical testing procedure, creating subgroups with insufficient numbers of patients, and ignoring the higher potential for chance differences to occur. Extrapolating the results selected from numerous subgroup analyses can be misleading if only selected differences are emphasized and others are ignored (see Chapter 17, Question 18).

d. Wrong statistical methods

The primary use of descriptive statistics is to describe the data clearly and concisely, while significance tests are designed to determine whether the differences detected between the experimental and control groups are real or due to chance. Poor extrapolation of the results can occur if the investigators use the wrong statistical methods to report the trial results. Description of the data can be misleading if the number of patients in the trial is small, the data are not properly classified, the distribution of the data departs significantly from normality, or statistical measures of centrality or variability are not used properly (see Chapter 17, Question 16). The results of significance tests can be misleading if they have low power, parametric tests are used with the wrong type of data, or multiple tests are used without guarding against the increased likelihood of Type I error. In addition, small but statistically significant differences between the experimental and control groups may improperly be considered clinically significant (see Chapter 17, Questions 18-20 and Chapter 18, Question 22).

e.   Selective reporting

The discussion of the reported results needs to cover all measures of drug efficacy and safety. Emphasis on only the positive results of the clinical drug trial may be misleading. In addition, problems such as protocol deviations and patient dropouts need to be evaluated for their potential impact on the extrapolation of the results. The presence of a significant number of protocol problems suggests a poor trial design or poor management of the trial participants. A significant participant dropout rate may result in important differences occurring between the trial patients and those who will receive the drug in clinical practice (see Chapter 17, Questions 14-15).

References

1.   Hamilton CW. How to write and publish scientific papers: scribing information for pharmacists. *Am J Hosp Pharm* 1992;49:2477-84.
2.   Walker AM.   Reporting the results of epidemiologic studies. *Am J Pub Health* 1986;76:556-8.
3.   Nahata MC. Publishing by pharmacists. *Drug Intell Clin Pharm* 1989;23:809-10.
4.   Kramer MS, Lane DA. Causal propositions in clinical research and practice. *J Clin Epidemiol* 1992;45:639-49.
5.   Maclure M.   Multivariate refutation of aetiological hypotheses in nonexperimental epidemiology. *Int J Epidemiol* 1990;19:782-7.
6.   Hutchinson TA, Lane DA. Standardized methods of causality assessment for suspected adverse drug reactions. *J Chron Dis* 1986;39:857-60.
7.   Gray-Donald K, Kramer MK. Causality inference in observational vs experimental studies. *J Epidemiol* 1988;127:885-93.
8.   Trout KS. How to read clinical journals: IV. To determine etiology or causation. *CMA Journal* 1981;124:985-90.
9.   Johnson JM. Reasonable possibility: causality and postmarketing surveillance. *Drug Info J* 1992;26:553-8.
10. Hill AB. Principles of medical statistics. Ninth ed. New York: Oxford University Press, 1971:309-27.
11. Greenland S. Randomization, statistics and causal inference. *Epidemiology* 1990;1:421-9.
13. Morton RF, Hebel JR, McCarter RJ. A study guide to epidemiology and biostatistics. Third ed. Rockville, MD: Aspen Press, 1990:35-46.
14. Koch GG, Hartzema AG. Basic statistical methods in pharmacoepidemiologic study designs. In Hartzema AG, Porta MS, Tilson HH, eds. Pharmacoepidemiology: an introduction. Cincinnati, OH: Harvey Whitney Books, 1990:142-75.
15. Browner WS, Newman TB. Are all significant p values created equal? *N Engl J Med* 1987;257:2459-63.
16. Koch GG, Sollecito WA. Statistical considerations in the design, analysis and interpretation of comparative clinical studies. *Drug Info J* 1984;18:131-51.
17. Oye RK, Shapiro MF. Reporting results from chemotherapy trials: does response make a difference in patient survival? *JAMA* 1984;252:2722-5.

18. Savitz D. Comments about statistical testing and confidence intervals. *Am J Pub Health* 1987;77:237-8.

19. Oxman AD, Guyatt GH. A consumer's guide to subgroup analysis. *Ann Intern Med* 1992;116:76-84.

20. Haunsperger DB, Saari DG. The lack of consistency for statistical decision procedures. *Am Stat* 1991;45:252-5.

21. O'Brien PC, Shampo MA. Statistics for clinicians: 6. Comparing two samples (the two-sample t test). *Mayo Clinic Proc* 1981;56:393-4.

22. Elenbaas RM, Elenbaas JK, Cuddy PG. Evaluating the medical literature, part II: statistical analysis. *Ann Emerg Med* 1983;12:610-20.

23. Gaddis GM, Gaddis ML. Introduction to biostatistics: part 3, sensitivity, specificity, predictive value and hypothesis testing. *Ann Emerg Med* 1990;19:591-7.

24. O'Brien PC, Shampo MA. Statistics for clinicians: epilogue. *Mayo Clinic Proc* 1981;56:755-6.

25. O'Brien PC, Shampo MA. Statistics for clinicians: 8. Comparing two proportions: the relative deviate test and chi-square equivalent. *Mayo Clin Proc* 1981;56:513-5.

26. Feinstein AR. Clinical Biostatistics I: a new name--and some other changes of the guard. *Clin Pharmacol Ther* 1970;11:135-148.

27. Pocock SJ. Basic principles of statistical analysis. In Pocock SJ, ed. Clinical trials: a practical approach. New York: J Wiley and Sons, 1983:188-209.

28. Sackett DL. How to read clinical journals: I. Why to read them and how to start reading them critically. *CMA Journal* 1981;124:555-8.

29. Hartzema AG. Guide to interpreting and evaluating the pharmacoepidemiologic literature. *Ann Pharmacother* 1992;26:96-8.

30. Pocock SJ. Current issues in the design and interpretation of clinical trials. *Br Med J* 1985;290:39-42.

31. Bailar JC, Mosteller F. Guidelines for statistical reporting in articles for medical journals. In Bailar JC and Mosteller F, eds. Medical use of statistics. Boston: NEJM books, 1992:313-331.

32. Ware JH, Mosteller F, Delgaudo F, Donnelly C, Ingelfinger JA. P values. In Bailar JC and Mosteller F, eds. Medical use of statistics. Boston: NEJM books, 1992:181-200.

33. Pocock SJ, Hughes MD. Estimation issues in clinical trials and overviews. *Stat Med* 1990;9:657-71.

34. Poole C. Beyond the confidence interval. *Am J Pub Health* 1987;77:195-9.

35. Thompson DW. Statistical criteria in the interpretation of epidemiologic data. *Am J Pub Health* 1987;77:191-4.

36. DeRuoen TA. Comments about statistical testing and confidence intervals. *Am J Pub Health* 1987;77:237.

37. Lachenbruch PA, Clark VA, Cumberland WG, Chang PC, Afifi AA, Flack VF, Elashoff RM. Comments about statistical testing and confidence intervals. *Am J Pub Health* 1987;77:237.

38. Fleiss JL. Significance tests have a role in epidemiologic research: reaction. *Am J Pub Health* 1987;76:559-60.

39. Subcutaneous Sumatriptan International Study Group. Treatment of migraine attacks with sumatriptan. *N Engl J Med* 1991;325:316-21.

40. Riegelman RK, Hirsch RP. Studying a study and testing a test: how to read the medical literature. 2nd ed. Boston: Little Brown, 1989.
41. Moses LE. Statistical concepts fundamental to investigations. In Bailar JC and Mosteller F, eds. Medical use of statistics. Boston: NEJM books, 1992:5-25.
42. Bailar JC. Some uses of statistical thinking. In Bailar JC and Mosteller F, eds. Medical use of statistics. Boston: NEJM books, 1992:27-44.
43. O'Connell JB, Mason JW. The applicability of results of streamlined trials to clinical practice: the myocarditis treatment trial. *Stat Med* 1990;9:193-7.
44. Murphy EA. Public and private hypotheses. *J Clin Epidemiol* 1989;42:79-84.
45. Bailar JC. Science, statistics, and deception. *Ann Intern Med* 1986;104:259-60.

SECTION IV   Appendices

Appendix A.   United States Drug Information Centers[a,b]

ALABAMA

Drug Information Service[a]
University of Alabama Hospital
619 South 19th Street
Birmingham, AL 35233
205-934-2162

Samford University Regional Drug[b]
Information Center
800 Lakeshore Boulevard
Birmingham, AL 35229
205-870-2891

ARIZONA

Arizona Poison and
Drug Information Center[a]
Arizona Health Sciences Center
1501 N. Campbell Avenue 3204K
Tucson, AZ 85724
602-626-6228

Tucson Medical Center
Drug Information Center
Department of Pharmacy
5301 East Grant Road
PO Box 42195
Tucson, AZ 85733
602-327-5461

ARKANSAS

Arkansas Poison and Drug
Information Center[a]
University of Arkansas for
Medical Sciences
4301 West Markham Street
Slot 522
Little Rock, AR 72205
501-686-5540

CALIFORNIA

Alta Bates-Herrick Hospital
Drug Information Service
3001 Colby Street
Berkeley, CA 94705
415-540-1503

Kaiser-Permanente
Drug Information Center
9521 Dalen Street
Downey, CA 90242
213-803-2940

Drug Information Analysis Center
Valley Medical Center
445 South Cedar Avenue
Fresno, CA 93702
209-453-4596

UCLA Medical Center
Drug Information Center
10833 LeConte Avenue
Los Angeles, CA 90024-1704
213-825-9755

Metropolitan State Hospital
Drug Information Center
11400 Norwalk Boulevard
Norwalk, CA 90650
213-863-7011 (Ext. 253, 237)

UCSD Drug Information Service
225 Dickinson Street H925
San Diego, CA 92103
619-294-6085

VA Medical - San Diego
3350 La Jolla Village Drive
c/o Department of Pharmacy
San Diego, CA 92161
611-552-8585 (Ext. 2422)

Drug Information Analysis
Service
University of California
San Francisco
Box 0622
San Francisco, CA 94143
415-476-4346

Western Medical Center/Santa Ana
1001 N. Tustin Avenue
Santa Ana, CA 92705
714-953-3398

Stanford University Medical Center
Department of Pharmacy
Room H0301
Stanford, CA 94305-2060
415-723-6422

COLORADO

The Kapoor Center for Pediatric
Drug Information
1056 East 19th Avenue, Box B-375
Denver, CO 80218
303-861-6835

Rocky Mountain Drug Consultation Center
Denver General Hospital
645 Bannock Street
Denver, CO 80204-4507
303-893-7774

Drug Information Service
University of Colorado
Health Science Center
Box C-239
4200 East 9th Avenue
Denver, CO 80262
303-270-8489

CONNECTICUT

University of Connecticut Health Center
Drug Information
Room C-2016
Farmington Avenue
Farmington, CT 06032
203-679-2782

Yale-New Haven Hospital
Drug Information Service[b]
20 York Street
New Haven, CT 06504
203-785-2248

DISTRICT OF COLUMBIA

Children's National Medical Center
Drug Information Center[a]
111 Michigan Avenue, N.W.
Washington, DC 20010
202-745-2055

Washington Hospital Center
110 Irving Street, N.W.
Washington, DC 20010
202-877-6646

FLORIDA

Drug Information and
Pharmacy Resource Center[b]
Box J316
J. Hillis Miller Health Center
Gainesville, FL 32610
904-395-0408

Drug Information Service[a,b]
University Medical Center
655 West 8th Street
Jacksonville, FL 32209
904-632-3995

Drug Information Center[b]
Jackson Memorial Hospital
Department of Pharmacy Service
1611 NW 12th Avenue
Miami, FL 33136
305-549-6898

UpFront Drug Information
5701 Biscayne Boulevard #602
Miami, FL 33137
305-757-2566

GEORGIA

Emory University
Drug Information Center
Emory University Hospital
1364 Clifton Road, NE
Atlanta, GA 30322
404-727-4644

Northside Hospital Pharmacy
Drug Information Service
1000 Johnson Ferry Road
Atlanta, GA 30342
404-851-8676

Medical College of Georgia
Drug Information Center
1120 15th Street
Augusta, GA 30912-5600
404-721-2887

IDAHO

Idaho Drug Information Service[b]
Pocatello Regional Medical Center
777 Hospital Way
Pocatello, ID 83201
208-236-0330

ILLINOIS

Drug Information Center
Northwestern Memorial Hospital
Superior Street and Fairbanks Court
Chicago, IL 60611
312-908-7573

St. Joseph Hospital
Drug Information Service[a,b]
Department of Pharmacy
2900 North Lake Shore Drive
Chicago, IL 60657
312-975-3199

Rush-Presbyterian-St. Luke's
Medical Center
Drug Information Center
1653 West Congress Parkway
Chicago, IL 60612
312-942-6525

University of Chicago Hospitals[b]
5841 South Maryland Avenue
Chicago, IL 60637
312-702-1388

University of Illinois Hospital
Drug Information Center
1740 West Taylor Street, Room C 300
M/C 883
Chicago, IL 60612
312-996-0209

Ingalls Memorial Hospital[b]
Drug Information Center
1 Ingalls Drive
Harvey, IL 60426
708-333-2300 (Ext. 4430)

Lutheran General Hospital
Drug Information Center
1775 Dempster
Park Ridge, IL 60068
708-696-8128

Northern Illinois Drug
Information Center[a]
Swedish American Hospital
1400 Charles Street
Rockford, IL 61108-1257
815-968-4400 (Ext. 4577)

INDIANA

Indiana University Hospitals
Drug Information Center
Pharmacy Department, UH N109A
926 West Michigan Street
Indianapolis, IN 46202-5271
317-274-3581

St. Vincent Hospital and
Health Care Center
2001 West 86th Street
Indianapolis, IN 46260
317-871-3200

IOWA

Mercy Hospital Medical Center
Drug Information Center[a]
Department of Pharmacy
6th and University Avenues
Des Moines, IA 50314
515-247-3286

Variety Club Poison and
Drug Information Center
Iowa Methodist Medical Center
1200 Pleasant Street
Des Moines, IA 50309
515-283-6254

Drug Information Service
Trinity Regional Hospital
Department of Pharmacy
Kenyon Road
Fort Dodge, IA 50501
515-573-7211

University of Iowa Hospitals
Drug Information Poison Control Center[a]
University of Iowa Hospital
Iowa City, IA 52242
319-356-2600

KANSAS

Kansas University Medical Center
39th & Rainbow Boulevard
Room B-400
Kansas City, KS 66103
913-588-2328

KENTUCKY

Drug Information Center
Chandler Medical Center
C-117 800 Rose Street
Lexington, KY 40536-0084
606-233-5320

LOUISIANA

St. Francis Medical Center[a]
309 Jackson Street
Monroe, LA 71201
318-362-4274

MARYLAND

Franklin Square Hospital Center[a]
9000 Franklin Square Drive
Baltimore, MD 21237
301-682-7700

The Johns Hopkins Hospital
Drug Information Center, Osler 527
600 North Wolfe Street
Baltimore, MD 21205
301-955-6348

University of Maryland
Drug Information Center[a]
20 North Pine Street, Room 201
Baltimore, MD 21201
410-328-7568

Pharmacy Department
Drug Information Center[a]
Memorial Hospital
Washington Street
Easton, MD 21601
301-822-1000 (Ext. 5645)

Drug Information Service
Pharmacy Department
Warren Magnuson Clinical Center
National Institutes of Health
Building 10, Room 1N-257
Bethesda, Maryland 20892
301-496-2407

MASSACHUSETTS

Brigham and Women's
Drug Information Center[b]
75 Francis Street
Boston, MA 02115
617-732-7166

Massachusetts Poison Control System[a]
300 Longwood Avenue
Boston, MA 02115
617-735-6609

Drug Information Center[b]
New England Medical Center
Pharmacy #420
750 Washington Street Box 420
Boston, MA 02111
617-956-5377

Drug Information Center
University of Massachusetts
Medical Center Hospital
55 Lake Avenue, North
Worcester, MA 01655
508-856-3456

MICHIGAN

University of Michigan
Drug Information Services
UHB2D301/0008
1500 E. Medical Center Drive
Ann Arbor, MI 48109-0008
313-936-8200

Harper Hospital
Drug Information Center
3990 John R.
Detroit, MI 48201
313-745-2006

Drug Information Center
Henry Ford Hospital
2799 West Grand Boulevard
Detroit, MI 48202
313-876-1229

Bronson Methodist Hospital[b]
Pharmacy Department
252 E. Lovell Street
Kalamazoo, MI 49007
616-341-7834

St. Joseph Mercy Hospital
Drug Information Center
900 Woodward Avenue
Pontiac, MI 48053
313-858-3050

Drug Information Center
Department of Pharmaceutical Services
William Beaumont Hospital
3601 West Thirteen Mile Road
Royal Oak, MI 48073
313-551-4077

Providence Hospital
Drug Information Center
16001 W. Nine Mile Road
Southfield, MI 48075
313-424-3121

MINNESOTA

University of Minnesota
Drug Information Services
3-160 Health Sciences Unit F
308 Harvard Street, SE
Minneapolis, MN 55455
612-624-9140

Saint Mary's Hospital
Mayo Medical Center
Pharmacy Department
Saint Mary's Hospital
1216 2nd Street S.W.
Rochester, MN 55902
507-285-5062

MISSISSIPPI

University of Mississippi
Drug Information Center
University Hospital
2500 North State Street
Jackson, MS 39212
601-984-2063

MISSOURI

St. John's Medical Center[a]
2727 McClelland Boulevard
Joplin, MO 64801
417-625-2452

UMKC Drug Information Center[b]
Truman Medical Center HG-C09
2301 Holmes Street
Kansas City, MO 64108
816-556-4125

St. Louis Drug Information Center[a,b]
St. Louis College of Pharmacy
4588 Parkview Place
St. Louis, MO 63110
314-454-8399

St. John's Drug Information and
Clinical Research Services
1235 East Cherokee Street
Springfield, MO 65804
417-885-3488

Western Missouri Medical Center
Pharmacy Department
Burkarth and East Gay Streets
Warrensburg, MO 64093
816-429-6434

NEBRASKA

Creighton University
Drug Information Service[b]
Health Science Library
Creighton University
California at 24th Street
Omaha, NE 68178
402-280-5101

Mid-Plains Poison Center[a]
8301 Dodge Street
Omaha, NE 68114
402-390-5555, 800-955-9119

University of Nebraska
Drug Information and
Education Services
600 South 42nd Street
Omaha, NE 68198-1090
402-559-4114

NEW JERSEY

New Jersey Poison/
Drug Information System
Newark Beth Israel Medical Center
201 Lyons Avenue
Newark, NJ 07112
201-926-7443

Drug Information Service
Department of Pharmacy
Robert Wood Johnson University Hospital
One Robert Wood Johnson Place
New Brunswick, NJ 08901
201-937-8842

The Valley Hospital[a]
223 N. Van Dien
Ridgewood, NJ 07450
201-447-8126

NEW MEXICO

New Mexico Poison and
Drug Information Center[a]
The University of New Mexico
Albuquerque, NM 87131-1076
505-277-4261 (administration)
505-843-2551 (service)

NEW YORK

Bronx Municipal Hospital
Center's Drug Information Center
Pelham Parkway South and
Eastchester Road
Bronx, NY 10461
212-918-4556

Montefiore Medical Center
Drug Information Center
111 E. 210th Street
Bronx, NY 10467
212-920-4511

International Drug Information Center[b]
A & M Schwartz College of Pharmacy
University Plaza
Brooklyn, NY 11201
718-403-1064

Drug Information Services
of Western New York
Pharmacy Department
462 Grider Street
Buffalo, NY 14215
716-898-3927

Mary Imogene Bassett Hospital
One Atwell Road
Cooperstown, NY 13326
607-547-3686

Lenox Hill Hospital
Drug Information Center[b]
100 E. 77th Street
New York, NY 10021
212-439-3190

Mount Sinai Medical Center
Drug Information Center
One Gustave L. Levy Place
New York, NY 10029
212-241-6619

The New York Hospital
Cornell Medical Center
Pharmacy Department, Room K-04
525 East 68th Street
New York, NY 10021
212-746-0740

Hudson Valley Poison Center[a]
Nyack Hospital
North Midland Avenue
Nyack, NY 10960
914-358-6200 (Ext. 2615)

University of Rochester
Drug Information Center[b]
601 Elmwood Avenue
Rochester, NY 14450
716-275-3718

Suffolk Drug Information Center
University Hospital
Pharmacy Department (L3 - Room 559)
SUNY at Stony Brook
Stony Brook, NY 11794
516-444-2672

NORTH CAROLINA

Drug Information Service
Manning Drive
University of North Carolina Hospitals
Chapel Hill, NC 27514
919-966-2373

Drug Information Service
Duke University Hospital
Box 3708
Durham, NC 27710
919-684-5125

The Triad Poison Center[a]
1200 North Elm Street
Greensboro, NC 27401-1020
919-379-4108

Pitt County Memorial Hospital
c/o East Carolina Drug Information
Center
200 Stantons Burg Road
Greenville, NC 27834
919-551-4257

Drug Information Service Center[b]
North Carolina Baptist Hospital
300 S. Hawthorne Road
Winston-Salem, NC 27103
919-748-2037

OHIO

Ohio Northern University
Drug Information Service[b]
Ada, OH 45810
419-772-2070

Drug and Poison Information Center[a,b]
University of Cincinnati
College of Medicine
231 Bethesda Avenue
Cincinnati, OH 45267-0144
513-558-5111

Cleveland Clinic Drug Information Center
9500 Euclid Avenue
Cleveland, OH 44195-5102
216-444-6456

Ohio State University Hospitals
410 West 10th Avenue
Columbus, OH 43210
614-293-8679

Bethesda Hospital
Drug Information Center[a]
Bethesda Hospital
2951 Maple Avenue
Zanesville, OH 43701
614-454-4300

OKLAHOMA

Presbyterian Hospital
Drug Information Center
N.E. 13th Street at Lincoln Boulevard
Oklahoma City, OK 73104
405-271-6226

University of Oklahoma
Drug Information Service[b]
1000 Stanton L. Young Boulevard
University of Oklahoma HSC
Oklahoma City, OK 73126
405-271-8080

Drug Information Service
St. Francis Hospital
6161 South Yale Avenue
Tulsa, OK 74136
918-494-6339

OREGON

University Drug Consultation Service[b]
Oregon Health Sciences University
3181 SW Sam Jackson Park Road
Portland, OR 97201
503-279-7530

PENNSYLVANIA

Geisinger Medical Center
Drug Information Service
Pharmacy 42-01
Danville, PA 17822-4201
717-271-8176

Hamot Medical Center[a]
201 State Street
Erie, PA 16550
814-870-6022

Thomas Jefferson University Hospital[b]
Drug Information Center
11th and Walnut Streets
Philadelphia, PA 19107
215-955-8877

Pharmacy and Drug Information
Hospital of the University of
Pennsylvania
3400 Spruce Street
Philadelphia, PA 19104
215-662-2900

Allegheny General Hospital
Drug Information Services
320 East North Avenue
Pittsburgh, PA 15212-9986
412-359-3192

Center for Drug Information[b]
Mercy Hospital of Pittsburgh
Duquesne University
School of Pharmacy
1400 Locust Street
Pittsburgh, PA 15219-5166
412-232-7903 (Ext. 7907)

Drug Information Center
Crozer-Chester Medical Center
1 Medical Center Boulevard
Upland, PA 19013
215-447-2851

Drug Information Center[b]
Williamsport Hospital and Medical Center
777 Rural Avenue
Williamsport, PA 17701
717-321-3289

PUERTO RICO

Centro de Informacion de
Medicamentos[b]
Escuela de Farmacia RCM
GPO Box 5067
San Juan, PR 00936
809-763-0196

RHODE ISLAND

URI Drug Information
Roger Williams Hospital
825 Chalkstone Avenue
Providence, RI 02908
401-456-2260

SOUTH CAROLINA

Drug Information Center[b]
Medical University of South Carolina
171 Ashley Avenue
Charleston, SC 29425
803-792-7527

Spartanburg Regional Medical Center
Drug Information Center
Spartanburg General Hospital
101 E. Wood Street
Spartanburg, SC 29301
803-591-6910

TENNESSEE

The University of Tennessee
Memorial Hospital
Pharmacy
1924 Alcoa Highway, Box 41
Knoxville, TN 37920
615-544-9125

University of Tennessee
Drug Information Center
210 Lamar Alexander Bldg.
877 Madison Avenue
Memphis, TN 38163
901-528-5555

TEXAS

Hermann Drug Information Center
Hermann Hospital
Department of Pharmaceutical Services
6411 Fannin Street
Houston, TX 77030
713-797-2073

M.D. Anderson Cancer Center
Drug Information Center
1515 Holcombe Boulevard
Houston, TX 77030
713-792-2858

The Methodist Hospital
Drug Information Center
6565 Fannin, DBI - 09
Houston, TX 77054
713-790-4190

Wilford Hall USAF Medical Center
Drug Information Center
Lackland AFB, TX 78236
512-670-5408

Methodist Hospital
Drug Information and Consultation Service
P.O. Box 1201
3615 19th Street
Lubbock, TX 79408
806-793-4012

UTAH

University of Utah Hospital
Drug Information Center[a]
Department of Pharmacy Services (A-050)
50 N. Medical Drive
Salt Lake City, UT 84132
801-581-2073

VIRGINIA

Medical College of Virginia Hospitals
Drug Information Center
Box 42, MCV Station
Richmond, VA 23298
804-786-0754

St. Mary's Hospital
Drug Information Center
5801 Bremo Road
Department of Pharmacy
Richmond, VA 23226
804-281-8058

WASHINGTON

Group Health Cooperative of
Puget Sound
801 SW 16th Street
Renton, WA 98057
206-235-3837

Washington State University
College of Pharmacy
West 601 First Avenue
Spokane, WA 99204-0399
509-456-4409

WISCONSIN

Drug Information Center
Department of Pharmacy Services
Meriter Hospital
202 S. Park Street
Madison, WI 53705
608-267-6084

University of Wisconsin Hospital
Drug and Poison Information Center
600 Highland Avenue
Madison, WI 53792
608-262-1315 (DI)
608-262-3702 (PI)

WYOMING

University of Wyoming
Drug Information Center
School of Pharmacy
Box 3375
Laramie, WY 82070
307-766-6128

Adapted with permission from Sandra L. Beaird, Pharm.D. and Rebecca M.R. Coley, M.S., R.Ph., St. Louis Drug Information Center, St. Louis, MO, 1991/92 Directory of Drug Information Centers.

[a]   Denotes centers which provide 24-hour service
[b]   Denotes centers which are fee-for-service

Appendix B.   Regional Canadian Drug Information Centers

British Columbia

British Columbia Drug and Poison
Information Centre (DPIC)
St. Paul's Hospital
1081 Burrard Street
Vancouver, British Columbia
Canada V6Z1Y6
604-682-2344 Ext. 2126

Alberta

PROVINCIAL POISON AND DRUG
INFORMATION SERVICE (PADIS)
Foothills Hospital
1403-29th Street NW
Calgary, Alberta T2N 2T9
403-670-1414 (Poison Information)
403-670-1222 (Drug Information)

Saskatchewan

DIAL ACCESS DRUG
INFORMATION SERVICE
University of Saskatchewan
Saskatoon, Saskatchewan S7N 0W0
306-966-6340

Consumer Drug Information Centre
(CDIC)
University of Saskatchewan
Saskatoon, Saskatchewan S7N 0W0
306-975-3784

Manitoba

Medication Information Line for the
Elderly (MILE)
Faculty of Pharmacy
University of Manitoba
Winnipeg, Manitoba R3T 2N2
204-261-3111

Ontario

METRODIS--Metro Toronto Hospitals
DI Service
Pharmacy Department
Sunnybrook Health Science Centre
2075 Bayview Avenue
North York, Ontario M4N 3M5
416-480-6100 Ext. 4514

OCP Drug Information Centre
Faculty of Pharmacy
University of Toronto
19 Russell Street
Toronto, Ontario M5S 2S2
416-978-4235

After September, 1992:
OCP Drug Information Centre
483 Huron Street
Toronto, Ontario M5R 2R4

OTTAWA VALLEY REGIONAL
DRUG INFORMATION SERVICE
(OVRDIS)
Pharmacy Department
Ottawa General Hospital
501 Smyth Road
Ottawa, Ontario K1H 8L6
613-737-8347

University Hospital Regional Drug
Information Service
(UH-LONDIS)
Department of Pharmacy Services
University Hospital
339 Windermere Road, Box 5339
London, Ontario, N6A 5A5
519-663-3172

Québec

CENTRE D'INFORMATION
PHARMAÇEUTIQUE (C.I.P.)
Hôpital du Sacré-Coeur de Montréal
5400, boul. Gouin ouest
Montréal, Québec H4J 1C5
514-338-2161

Hôpital General Juif-Sir
Mortimer B. Davis (Jewish General)
3755 Chemin de la Côte Ste. Catherine,
Montréal, Québec H3T 1E2
514-340-8222 ext. 4671

Nova Scotia/New Brunswick/PEI

Regional Drug Information Service
(RDIS)
Camp Hill Medical Centre
1763 Robie Street
Halifax, Nova Scotia B3H 3G2
902-496-2211

Adapted with permission from *Can J Hosp Pharm* 1992;45:79-85. This information is current as of February 1992. For the most recent listing, please contact the Canadian Society of Hospital Pharmacists, 1145 Hunt Club Road, Suite 350, Ottawa, Ontario, Canada K1V 0Y3 Phone: 613-736-9733 Fax: 613-736-5660.

Appendix C.   European Drug Information Centers

AUSTRIA

Osterreichische Apothekerkammer
Spitalgasse 31, Postfach 87
A 1091 Vienna, Austria

Tel: 0222/4256 76/203
Telex: 114366 apkam

BELGIUM

A.P.B. Service de Documentation
Scientifique Documentatiedienst
Rue Archimede 11
B-1040, Brussels, Belgium

Tel: 02/230.26.85
Telex: 61833

Ministere de la Sante Publique et de
l'Environnement
Inspection Generale de la Pharmacie
cite Administrative de l'Etat Quartier
Vesale,
1010 Brussels, Belgium

Tel: 02/210.49.04 - 210.49.05
Telex: 25768 MUGSPFF B

DENMARK

DAK Laboratories
P.O. Box 1911
Leorgravsvej 59
DK-2300 Copenhagen, Denmark

Tel: 01551188
Telefax: 01589688

FRANCE

Pharmacie Centrale
Center De Documentation et
D'Information
Hopitaux de Paris
7 Rue Du Fer A Moulin
BP O9, 75221 Paris, France

Tel: 33(1)47070220/43371100
Telex: 204 203 F Pharmap
Fax: 33(1)43379597

GERMANY

Bundesvereiningung Deutscher
Apothekerverbande-ABDA
P.O. Box 970108
D-6000 Frankfurt 97, Germany

Tel: 069 7544-1 (-243/244)
Telex: 414804

IRELAND

Pharmaceutical Society of Ireland
37 Northumberland Road
Ballsbridge, Dublin 4, Ireland

Tel: 0001 600699 and 0001
         600551

School of Pharmacy
Trinity College Dublin
18 Shrewsbury Road
Dublin 4, Ireland

Tel: 0001 693212

IRELAND continued

National Drugs Advisory Board
Charles Lucas House
63-64 Adelaide Road
Dublin 2, Ireland

Tel: 0001 764971/7
Telex: 90542

Pharmacy Department
Beaumont Hospital
Beaumont Road,
Dublin 9, Ireland

Tel: 0001 377755 (Ext. 2840)
Telex: 33353 BHB E1

Drug Information Center
St. James's Hospital
Dublin 8, Ireland

Tel: 0001 537941 (Ext. 2554)

Pharmacy Department
St. Vincents Hospital
Elm Park,
Dublin 4, Ireland

Tel: 0001 694533 (Ext. 4284)

ITALY

SRLRD/Scientific Information
Department
Via C Imbonati, 24
20153 Milan, Italy

Tel: 2 6335 314
Telex: 330314 ERBA 1

S. Quattrocchi
Via Furipide 1
20145 Milan, Italy

Tel: 02 4395009
Fax: 02 4395125

Marino Necri Pharmacological Research
Institute
Via Eritrea 62
20157 Milan, Italy

Tel: 02 357941
Telex: 33 1268

Centro Regionale di Informazione
Sul Farmaco
Servizio Farmaceutico U.S.S.L.
Via San Francoesco da Paola 31
Torino 1, Italy

Tel: 0039/11/8398506
Fax: 8122492

Centro Di Documentazione E,
Informazione Sul Farmaco
c/o Farmacia Ospedale Polidimis
Borgoroma, 34100 Verona, Italy

Tel: 045 584490 933613
Fax: 045 584490

NETHERLANDS

P.A.G.M. de Smet
Drug Information Center
Alexanderstraat 11
2514 JL The Hague
The Netherlands

Tel: 070 3624111

Klinische Formacie
Documentatie en Informatie
Geert Grooteplein Z 8
Postbus 9101, 6500 HB Nijmegen
The Netherlands

Tel: 3180515120

NORWAY

Department of Pharmacotherapeutics
University of Oslo, POB 1065 Blindern
N-0316, Oslo, Norway

Tel: 47 2 45050/56 or 694265
Fax: 47 2 695401

PORTUGAL

CEDIME (Centro de Documentaçáo e
Informaçáo de Medicamentos)
Pc Principe Real 18,
1200 Lisboa, Portugal

Tel: 323821/47/54
Telex: 42666

SPAIN

Consejo General de Colegios Oficiales de
Farmaceuticos
Villanueva, 11
28001 Madrid, Spain

Tel: 91 2763903 4312560 (Ext. 212)
Telex: 91 2763905

SWEDEN

Apoteksbolaget
S-105114 Stockholm, Sweden

Tel: 08 7839650
Fax: 08 7805817
Telex: 11553

SWITZERLAND

CHUV Center Hospitalier Universitaire
Vaudois, Pharmacie,
CH-1011 Lausanne, Switzerland

Tel: 021 41 11 11 41 34 64
Telex: 455012 chuv ch

Documentation Galencia
Untermatt Leig 8,
CH-3001 Bern, Switzerland

Tel: 031 553033
Telex: 911791

UNITED KINGDOM

London (North East Thames)

Regional Drug Information Center
The London Hospital
Whitechapel,
London, E1 1BB, England

Tel: 01 247 5976
        01 377 7489 (direct line)
Fax: 01 377 7122 (call 7123)

Cardiff (Wales)

Welsh Drug Information Center
University Hospital of Wales
Heath Park,
Cardiff, CF4 4XW, Wales

Tel: 0222 755944 (Ext. 2979, 2251)
        0222 759541 (direct line)
Fax: 0222 752645

Northern Ireland (Belfast)

Regional Drug and Poison Information
Service
Royal Victoria Hospital
Belfast, BT12 6BA,
Northern Ireland

Tel: 0232 240503 (Ext. 2032, 3847)
        0232 248095 (direct line)

Scotland (Edinburgh)

Drug Information Center
Royal Infirmary of Edinburgh
Lauriston Place,
Edinburgh, EH3 9YW
Scotland

Tel: 031 229 2477 (Ext. 2094, 2416,
        2443)
        031 229 3901 (direct line)
Fax: 031 228 5402

Adapted with permission from Maguire ME, D'Arcy PF. Present drug information services in Europe including 'The two pharmacists of Verona'. *Int Pharm J* 1990;4:49-56.

Appendix D.   Forms for Reporting Adverse Drug Reactions and Drug Product Problems: FDA Form 3500 and USP Drug Product Problem Reporting Form

FDA Form 3500

USP Drug Product Problem Reporting Form

USP PRACTITIONERS' REPORTING NETWORK[SM]
An FDA MEDWATCH *partner*

DRUG PRODUCT •PROBLEM•

REPORTING PROGRAM

1. PRODUCT NAME (brand name and generic name)

2. DOSAGE FORM (tablet, capsule, injectable, etc.)	3. SIZE/TYPE OF CONTAINER	4. STRENGTH	5. NDC NUMBER

6. LOT NUMBER(S)	7. EXPIRATION DATE(S)

8. NAME AND ADDRESS OF THE MANUFACTURER	9. NAME AND ADDRESS OF LABELER (if different from manufacturer)

10. YOUR NAME & TITLE (please type or print)

11. YOUR PRACTICE LOCATION (include establishment name, address and zip code)

Days and times available _____

12. PHONE NUMBER AT PRACTICE LOCATION (include area code)

14a. If requested, will the actual product involved be available for examination by the manufacturer or FDA? *(Do not send samples to USP.)* ☐ Yes ☐ No

13. PLEASE INDICATE TO WHOM USP MAY VOLUNTARILY DISCLOSE YOUR IDENTITY
You may release my identity to: (check box[es] that apply)

☐ The manufacturer and/or labeler as listed above ☐ The Food and Drug Administration ☐ Other persons requesting a copy of this report

b. Date problem occurred or observed: _____

c. This event has been reported to: ☐ Manufacturer ☐ FDA

Other _____

15. SIGNATURE OF REPORTER	16. DATE

17. PROBLEMS NOTED OR SUSPECTED (if more space is needed, please attach separate page)

Return To:
USP PRN[SM]
12601 Twinbrook Parkway
Rockville, Maryland 20852

Call or FAX Toll Free:
1-800-4-USP PRN

File Access Number:

Date Received by USP:

Date Firm Notified:

Additional forms can be found in the USP DI Vol. I and Vol. III and in all monthly Updates.

Appendix E.   Supplemental Standards and Learning Objectives for Residency Training in Drug Information Practice of the American Society of Hospital Pharmacists

---

Preamble

Definition. A specialized residency in drug information practice is defined as a postgraduate program of organized education and training that meets the requirements set forth and approved by the American Society of Hospital Pharmacists. The ASHP Accreditation Standard for Specialized Residency Training[1] together with this supplement, are the basic criteria used to evaluate drug information residency training programs in institutions applying for accreditation by the American Society of Hospital Pharmacists.

A specialized residency in drug information practice must be organized and conducted to develop a mastery of knowledge and an expert level of competency in this area of pharmacy, differentiated in scope, depth, and proficiency from the drug information activities of institutional pharmacy residents. Objectives of such training shall include extensive experiences in providing comprehensive drug information services in an institution or with several institutions, integrated with the institution's clinical pharmacy services, drug-distribution systems, and the appropriate committees dealing with drug use.

Qualifications of the Training Site. The parent facility for an accredited residency in drug information pharmacy practice shall be a general hospital or a health science center that is formally affiliated with one or more general hospitals.

Two or more hospitals may collaborate in conducting a drug information residency program, provided that one hospital is identified as the primary site and one individual is designated as the residency program director.

Qualifications of the Pharmacy Service. The pharmacy department in which an accredited drug information practice residency is based must meet the requirements set forth in Standard II of the ASHP Accreditation Standard for Specialized Pharmacy Residency Training.[1] In addition, the pharmacy department must provide a comprehensive program of drug information services far beyond that required in the ASHP Minimum Standard for Pharmacies in Institutions.[2] The following specific requirements are established for the drug information service program.

Physical Facilities. There shall be a defined area for the drug information center. Space shall be adequate to house the furniture, equipment, literature resources, and personnel of the drug information center.

Resources. There shall be a comprehensive drug information library with appropriate holdings of primary, secondary, and tertiary literature. Scientific and professional practice journals in pharmacy and medicine shall be available in the drug information center or quickly accessible in another location. At least two secondary information services (indexing or abstracting services) shall be available in the drug information center. Reference texts shall be current and provide detailed information in at least the following areas of drug information: administration, adverse effects, availability, bioavailability, chemistry, cost, dose, drugs of choice, efficacy, excretion, formulations, incompatibilities, identifications (foreign and American), indications, interactions, laws, mechanisms of action, nonprescription drugs, pathophysiology, pharmacokinetics, statistics, teratogenicity, tissue distribution, and toxicology.

The drug information center should be located near a medical library that, in turn, has access to a regional medical library.

Computer-search capabilities shall be available in the drug information center or through the medical library.

Staffing. At least one full-time drug information specialist shall be employed in the drug information center. Secretarial and clerical support shall be readily available to the drug information center staff, including typing of communications, filing, and related duties.

Availability of Service. The drug information center shall be open for service at least eight hours per day, Monday through Friday, with off-hours service capability through a paging system, answering service, or other mechanism.

Scope of Service. The drug information service program shall be oriented toward patient-specific requests, and it shall respond to at least five (minimum average) such requests per day. Documentation of all responses shall be maintained. The drug information center shall also provide the following services on a regular basis: development of drug monographs for use by the pharmacy and therapeutics committee, participation in ongoing drug-use review and medical audits, publication of therapeutics newsletters, and formal instruction of students or residents. The following additional services should be provided where feasible: investigational drug information clearinghouse, adverse drug reaction reporting, drug information support service to other institutions, and formulary revision.

Location. Drug information centers located outside the pharmacy department (e.g., a medical library or college of pharmacy) may be used as training sites, provided that they meet the requirements set forth in this section (Qualifications of the Pharmacy Service) and are routinely used in the hospital pharmacy's drug information service program.

Qualifications of the Preceptor. The area of specialization of the preceptor shall be drug information pharmacy practice. He shall have had a minimum of three years of experience operating a drug information center. In addition, he shall maintain an active patient-care involvement, either through clinical consultations and other patient-oriented services provided through the drug information center or through other routinely provided clinical pharmacy services

Qualifications of the Applicant. In addition to meeting the requirements set forth in Standard IV, the applicant should have completed formal academic instruction in the following subject areas or their equivalents: drug-literature evaluation, pathophysiology, statistics, and toxicology.

The following learning objectives shall be approved by the Commission on Credentialing following review annually by a committee appointed from the Special Interest Group on Drug and Poison Information Practice of the American Society of Hospital Pharmacists.

Learning Objectives and Areas of Emphasis

I.   **Learning Objectives.** A resident who completes an accredited program in drug information practice shall be able to:
  A.   Develop a plan for the organization and operation of a drug information service, including physical accommodations, reference sources, professional and supportive personnel, budgeting, relationships with other health-care departments, work flow, assumed or designated responsibilities, and documentation of services.
  B.   Make effective use of institutional and extramural library facilities and librarian services.
  C.   Select the most appropriate drug information literature sources for any given question.
  D.   Use the primary literature, including the pharmacy practice literature, in providing drug information services.
  E.   Demonstrate a mastery of drug information filing systems.
  F.   Evaluate written and verbal promotional material about drugs provided by pharmaceutical representatives.
  G.   Apply a knowledge of biopharmaceutics in selecting drug products and in solving patient-specific drug-therapy problems.
  H.   Evaluate the study design of research articles in the drug literature, and state an opinion on the validity of the published results.
  I.   Communicate effectively, in person and by telephone, with pharmacists, nurses, physicians, patients, and pharmaceutical representatives in solving drug information problems.
  J.   Obtain appropriate patient, drug, and disease information from an inquirer initiating a patient-oriented drug information request.
  K.   Write concise, authoritative, grammatically correct, and clinically applicable consultations, drug monographs, and other drug-related manuscripts.

L. Respond to patient-specific inquiries in time for maximum clinical usefulness.

M. Provide rapid and accurate information relating to poison treatment.

N. Respond with authority to questions relating to drug-induced disorders.

O. Provide a pharmacy and therapeutics committee with drug information support, including comparative drug-monograph reviews.

P. Take charge of the organization, preparation, and dissemination of an in-house periodic bulletin or newsletter (e.g., drug information bulletin/newsletter. pharmacy and nursing newsletter, or P&T committee newsletter).

Q. Contribute to the practice of pharmacy-based drug information services through publication of a therapeutic review, drug monograph, case report, or the results of original research.

R. Make a clear statement about the organization and role of a hospital's institutional review board, the relationship of the pharmacist to its activities, and the role of the pharmacist in distribution and control of investigational drugs.

S. Initiate a drug-use review or medical audit.

T. Participate in the formal inservice training or continuing education of physicians, pharmacists, nurses, or other health-care professionals in therapeutic areas, and conduct classes and training sessions dealing with drug information skills and knowledge for appropriate groups of learners.

U. Develop and defend a proposal for implementing a research project or a new drug information service or other clinical service.

V. Participate in research activities that include, but are not restricted to, clinical and preclinical drug studies, surveillance of clinical drug experiences in the institution, evaluation of new and innovative services, and drug-use review.

II. **Areas of Emphasis**. The resident's training program shall be structured around practical applications of drug-literature retrieval and analysis in solving clinical problems, and associated communications skills. It must be organized in a way that makes possible the attainment of the learning objectives. Experiences must be provided in each of the following areas:

A. *Use of drug information literature.*

1. Primary literature (journals). The resident must receive extensive experience in the use of journals in pharmacy, medicine, and the pharmaceutical and biomedical sciences

2. Secondary sources. The resident must have an expert knowledge in the use of at least two of the following sources and be capable of using the others when necessary: Current Contents, de Haen Drugs in Research, de Haen Drugs in Use, Index Medicus, Inpharma, Iowa Drug Information Service, International Pharmaceutical Abstracts, Reactions, and Science Citation Index. Skill in using the following special information systems is also expected: Drugdex, Poisindex, and Unlisted Drugs.

3. Tertiary literature (reference books). The resident must have experience in using current, standard textbooks or reference volumes in solving drug information problems. The resident's experience should include use of books in each of the following subject areas: adverse effects, administration, availability, bioavailability, chemistry, drug cost, dose, drugs of choice, efficacy, excretion, formulations, incompatibilities, identifications (foreign and American), indications, interactions, laws, mechanism of action, nonprescription drugs, pathophysiology, pharmacokinetics, statistics, teratogenicity, tissue distribution, and toxicology.

B. *Drug-induced (iatrogenic) disease.* The resident shall receive instruction and training in evaluating the pathophysiology, mechanism of action, and treatment of drug induced disorders.

C. *Toxic drug ingestion.* The resident shall receive instruction and training in evaluating potentially toxic drug ingestions and providing information to patients and to other health professionals concerning signs and symptoms, general supportive care, and specific treatment.

D. *Information storage.* The resident shall receive training in proper storage (filing) of special drug information, such as formulation contents of pharmaceuticals and drug distribution to specialized body compartments.

E. *Communications skills.* The resident shall have numerous assignments throughout the year aimed at developing written and verbal communications skills. The residency preceptor shall be specifically responsible for setting goals for the resident's growth and development in these areas, monitoring the resident's progress, and counseling the resident on a regular basis concerning communication abilities.

F. *Clinical practice skills.* The resident shall have adequate experiences throughout the year to maintain a good level of expetise in clinical practice.

Extramural Experiences

When appropriate, rotations or visitations to other institutions should be scheduled to augment the resident's training (e.g., a poison control center, a pharmacokinetics consultation service, a federal drug information agency, a pharmaceutical company information center, and a medical library or pharmacy school information center). If the drug information service does not answer poison information inquiries, a rotation in a poison control center shall be required. Special rotations may also be arranged to strengthen the resident's clinical, communications, and research skills.

Extramural rotations may be conducted either as full-time training activities (e.g., a one-month block), or on a regularly scheduled part-time basis. If extramural rotations are scheduled for the purpose of pursuing one or more of the fundamental learning objectives, there must be a pharmacist preceptor who has defined responsibilities for monitoring the progress and evaluating the accomplishments of the resident. A detailed set of objectives for extramural rotations must be prepared in advance. The qualifications of the extramural training site are subject to review and approval by the American Society of Hospital Pharmacists.

Research Projects

The residency training schedule shall make provision for the resident's participation in a self-directed or collaborative research project. The final report of the project should be of such quality to merit presentation at a national professional meeting or publication in an appropriate journal.

References

1.   American Society of Hospital Pharmacists. ASHP accreditation standard for specialized pharmacy residency training (with guide to interpretation). *Am J Hosp Pharm* 1980;37:1229-32.
2.   American Society of Hospital Pharmacists. ASHP minimum standard for pharmacies in institutions. *Am J Hosp Pharm* 1977;34:1356-8.

Approved by the ASHP Board of Directors. September 24, 1982. The initial draft was developed by a working group of the SIG on Drug and Poison Information Pharmacy Practice. The final document was approved by the Commission on Credentialing before submission to the Board of Directors.

Reprinted with permission from the *American Journal of Hospital Pharmacy* 1982;39:1970-2.

Appendix F.   Quality Assurance Guidelines for Responding to Drug Information Questions

---

I. Demographic data: complete
    A. Full name and telephone number were present.
    B. Location, profession, preparation time, and formal written consultation were indicated.
    C. Date received, time received, time needed, and person who received the question (initials are sufficient) were indicated.
    D. Address was present if written response was needed.
II. Background information
    A. Appropriate: for patient-specific requests, information was obtained for pertinent (not necessarily all) medications, dosages, disease states, and laboratory values.
    B. Comprehensive: sufficient information was documented so reviewer has a clear idea why request was made.
III. Ultimate question
    A. Clear: it is evident what was searched.
    B. Concise: the ultimate question was direct and succinct.
IV. Search strategy
    A. Relevant: references likely to provide useful information were used in the search.
    B. Comprehensive: all pertinent references were used in the search.
    C. Reference format
        1. Written consultations: all resources were referenced according to the Uniform Requirements for Manuscripts Submitted to Biomedical Journals (*Ann Intern Med* 1988;108:258-65; updated version: *JAMA* 1993;269:2282-6).
        2. Oral consultations:
            a. Journal article: Uniform Manuscript Requirements.
            b. Textbook: title, year or edition, and page number.
            c. Computerized drug consultations: title, consultation number, and date.
            d. Secondary reference: title, date, and page number.
            e. Contact person: name, title, phone number, and date.
        3. Personal knowledge: it is acceptable to respond to a request based on personal knowledge, but the response is subject to verification by the quality assurance reviewer. Therefore, the responder must be sure that the information can be substantiated by the literature.
V. Literature retrieved
    A. Evaluation: the responder synthesized and evaluated (not merely summarized) the data from various sources to form a logical and coherent conclusion.
    B. Documentation: all data used to answer the request were footnoted.
VI. Response
    A. Accurate: response was correct and supported by the literature that was retrieved and documented.
    B. Objective: response was unbiased and based on the literature evaluated; opinions were clearly separated from facts.
    C. Complete: the search was sufficiently comprehensive so that all relevant issues pertaining to the request were addressed.
    D. Timely: a response was provided within the time frame determined at the initiation of the request. If a complete response could not be provided within this time, preliminary information was provided to the caller within the time frame, with follow-up when all data were gathered. Time of all follow-up calls was noted on the request form. Written responses to all nonpatient questions were mailed within two weeks of the date of the request. Written responses to patient-specific questions were mailed within one week.

Adapted with permission from Restino MSR, Knodel LC. Drug information quality assurance program used to appraise students' performance. *Am J Hosp Pharm* 1992;49:1425-9.

Appendix G.   Rating Scales for Quality Assurance Evaluation of Drug Information
Responses

Judgmental Responses

These responses represent the highest degree of sophistication and require judgment. A formal written response is usually required, although oral responses may suffice for some requests. Integration of new data with pre-existing knowledge and experience is required. In addition to extensive searching of tertiary and secondary references, a primary literature review is usually required. For judgmental drug information requests that are patient-specific, detailed information pertaining to the patient's clinical condition is essential. Examples of judgmental drug information requests are drug therapy evaluation and recommendations, identification and attribution of adverse drug reactions, and complex dosage adjustments based on pharmacokinetics, disease state, or drug interactions.

5   The response was excellent, comprehensive, and well written (if applicable). An in-depth literature search was required, with synthesis and analysis of data that are not readily accessible in comprehensive reference textbooks. This level is expected for most written consultations and for some complex oral consultations.
4   The consultation was very good, but a minor problem with documentation, comprehensiveness, timeliness, writing, or other important aspect existed.
3   This is the minimum acceptable level for judgmental responses. The consultation was good, but minor problems with documentation, comprehensiveness, timeliness, writing, or other important aspect existed.
2   Significant deficiencies with regard to documentation, comprehensiveness, timeliness, writing, or other important aspect of the consultation existed, but the response was basically adequate.
1   Significant deficiencies made the consultation unacceptable for use. The response was incorrect, inadequate, biased, poorly written, or poorly documented.

Nonjudgmental Responses

These responses represent a lower degree of sophistication and do not require judgment. Oral responses are usually adequate, although written responses sometimes may be required. Extensive searching of tertiary, secondary, and primary references is not commonly required, since these requests often can be answered from general knowledge or standard textbooks. Nonjudgmental requests are usually not patient-specific. Examples of nonjudgmental requests are drug identification, availability or cost, compatibility or stability, physical characteristics, pharmacokinetics (absorption, distribution, metabolism, elimination), or teratogenicity and lactation.

5   The response was excellent, comprehensive, well-documented, and timely. For some questions, an integration of data obtained from several references may be necessary to formulate a response.
4   Other than a minor problem with documentation, comprehensiveness, timeliness, or other important aspect, the response was very good.
3   This is the minimum acceptable level for nonjudgmental responses. The response was good, but problems with documentation, comprehensiveness, timeliness, or other important aspect existed.
2   Significant deficiencies with regard to documentation, comprehensiveness, timeliness, or other important aspect existed, but the response was basically adequate.
1   Significant deficiencies made the consultation unacceptable for use. The response was inadequate, incorrect, biased, or poorly documented.

Reprinted with permission from Restino MSR, Knodel LC. Drug information quality assurance program used to appraise students' performance. *Am J Hosp Pharm* 1992;49:1425-9.

Appendix H.   Sample Drug Information Data Collection Form

DRUG INFORMATION DATA COLLECTION FORM

Date _____ Time _____ Receiver_____ Responder_____

DEMOGRAPHIC DATA
Requestor:_____ Dept/Affiliation_____
Phone/Pager:_____ Location/City_____
Profession: __MD/DO __RN __PA/NP __Student __DDS/DMD
          __RPh/PharmD __Other:_____

INITIAL QUESTION

BACKGROUND INFORMATION
(age, sex, weight, disease states, medications, lab values, allergies, etc.)

ULTIMATE QUESTION

Classification (check only one category):
__Availability (strength, manufacturer, formulary)   __Pharmacokinetics
__Compatibility/Stability/Administration (rate/method)   __Laws/Policy & Procedure/P&T
__Therapy Evaluation/Drug of Choice   __Adverse Effects
__Identification   __Teratogenicity/Genetic Effects
__Drug Interactions (drug, lab, disease, food)   __Poisoning/Toxicology
__Dosage/Regimen Recommendations   __Cost
__General Product Information   __Lactation/Infant Risks
__Pharmaceutics (compounding, formulations)   __Foreign/Investigational
__Referral: __pharmacokinetics __poison control __nutrition __library ___ other:_____

SEARCH STRATEGY
(indicate resource and utility [+ or -]; record specific data on back)

_____   _____   _____

FINDINGS/EVALUATION/RESPONSE

Responder/Supervisor_____/_____ Written Response: ___Y ___N Date____/___/____
Time___:___ Time spent:_____

FOLLOW-UP INFORMATION
(note attempts to contact, messages left) _____

Adapted with permission from the Medical College of Virginia Drug Information Service

Appendix I.   Sample Written Consultations

Jon A. Doe, M.D., University Hospital   October 3, 1993

Dear Dr. Doe,

I am sorry I was not able to answer your returned phone call last Friday, March 15. My colleague, Jane Smith, informed me that you would like a written response to your question regarding adverse reactions to iron dextran administration.

Your patient appeared to experience a typical delayed-type reaction which has been reported to occur in 5-15% of patients after IV or IM administration of large doses of iron dextran. These reactions generally commence 24-48 hours after administration and can include arthralgias, chills, fever, malaise, etc. Resolution of symptoms is complete, but may require 3-4 days, or 3-7 days, after iv or im administration, respectively. I refer you to two references (copies included) which describe this type of reaction and the temporal relationships (Imferon® Package Insert, Fisons Corporation, Bedford, MA; Iron Dextran Injection monograph, Drug Information 90, American Society of Hospital Pharmacists, Bethesda, MD 1990:714-6).

Delayed adverse effects have been reported after both im and iv administration, and there are insufficient data to draw conclusions regarding the relative safety of these routes.

Development of delayed adverse effects that are not life-threatening is not a contraindication to further treatment with iron dextran. In fact, in one large series of cases (Hamstra RD, et al. *JAMA* 1980;243:1726-31), the authors found that in some patients subsequent reactions were often less severe than the initial one. The authors reported the details of several patients who received multiple injections after experiencing reactions and I would suggest this as a good source for information regarding repeated administration.

Pretreatment with antihistamines, such as chlorpheniramine 4 mg or diphenhydramine 50 mg, 30 minutes before administration appears to be helpful in preventing or reducing the severity of the reactions. Dilution of iron dextran in normal saline may reduce the phlebitis that has been associated with administration in D5W solutions. Doses of less than 250 mg may be less likely to cause adverse effects.

I hope this information is helpful. If I can be of further assistance, please contact me or anyone in the Drug Information Service at ext. 1234.

John L. Smith, Pharm.D.
Drug Information Specialist   enclosures (3)

Adapted using pseudonyms with permission from the Medical College of Virginia Drug Information Service.

Memorandum

DATE: April 10, 1993

TO: Joseph P. Brown, M.D.
            Rehabilitation, Box 222

FROM: Mary F. Thomas, Pharm.D.
            Drug Information Service
            Box 15, Community Hospital

RE: Livedo Reticularis Associated with Amantadine Use

In follow up to our conversation regarding the mechanism and contributing factors for livedo reticularis during amantadine treatment, I am providing two references[1,2] which characterize this common side effect and provide some of the details you have been seeking. Vollum and colleagues compared the occurrence and extent of livedo reticularis in 40 patients with Parkinson's disease receiving amantadine 100-400 mg per day for 2 to 12 months (mean 11 months) versus 51 control patients not having Parkinson's disease. Of the treated patients, 36 of 40 had livedo, spontaneously reported by 16 patients, versus 32 of 51 controls, most of whom had not noticed the network pattern of skin discoloration. In treated patients livedo was not associated with higher dosages of amantadine; livedo became more pronounced on the lower extremities when the patients were standing. Twenty of 36 patients with livedo had some degree of ankle edema. While ankle edema was not seen in the absence of livedo, the severity of ankle edema was not directly related to the severity of livedo. Based on clinical and laboratory examinations and skin biopsies, there was no evidence of any drug-related systemic disease process in the amantadine treated patients with livedo. When amantadine was discontinued in three patients, livedo gradually disappeared over 6 to 12 weeks. The investigators proposed that livedo reticularis in patients receiving amantadine is a physiologic response to drug-induced catecholamine depletion in peripheral nerve endings; it is not a pathologic process resulting from arteritis affecting dermal vessels as is seen in drug-induced lupus erythematosus or some other systemic diseases. Schwab and colleagues conclude that livedo reticularis in patients receiving amantadine has no therapeutic significance, other than cosmetic consequences, and does not require that therapy be interrupted.

Enclosures (2)
References:
1. Vollum DI, Parkes JD, Doyle D. Livedo reticularis during amantadine treatment. *Br Med J* 1971;2:627-8.
2. Schwab RS, Poskanzer DC, England AC, Young RR. Amantadine in Parkinson's disease. *JAMA* 1972;222:792-5.

John B. Allen, M.D., Adult Allergy Clinic   June 7, 1993

Dear Dr. Allen:

In follow-up to your request on May 25, 1993, regarding the availability of tetanus toxoid fluid for use as an intradermal skin test, I have included an article which may be of interest. Jacobs and colleagues[1] retrospectively reviewed 740 charts of patients with a history of reaction to tetanus toxoid immunization. The purpose of this study was to determine any correlation between the response to a tetanus toxoid challenge and the history of adverse reaction, the skin test response, or the interval from last immunization. Intradermal skin tests were performed using serial tenfold-dilutions of commercially prepared plain tetanus toxoid. If there was no response to the 1:100 v/v intradermal test, a subcutaneous challenge was begun using diphtheria and tetanus toxoids, adsorbed. Seven-hundred thirty of 740 patients were non-reactive to skin testing and subcutaneous tetanus toxoid challenge. Of the 95 patients who originally reported anaphylactoid symptoms, 94 had a negative response to the skin test and tolerated the challenge doses without a reaction. One patient with previous anaphylactoid symptoms had an immediate skin reaction to intradermal testing, but tolerated a full immunizing tetanus dose without adverse effects. Another patient, who previously experienced a syncopal episode with immunization, reacted to the skin testing, but later tolerated a full challenge.

The authors concluded that prior history of adverse reaction to tetanus toxoid poorly correlated with subsequent reactions to skin testing and immunization. They also noted the poor correlation between intervals since last immunization and subsequent response. Thus, the authors claimed that a history of adverse reaction to tetanus toxoid should not preclude future immunizations. Three patients demonstrated hypersensitivity to mercury, which is found as a preservative (thimerosal), in tetanus toxoid fluid and in diphtheria and tetanus toxoids, adsorbed. It was decided that the use of tetanus and diphtheria immunizations should not be avoided due to mercury sensitivity, as only local cell-mediated (Type IV) hypersensitivity is expected and can be treated.

Results indicate that reactions to tetanus toxoid are rare. Even those patients who did react to skin testing were able to tolerate full immunization doses without adverse effects. Thus it seems that history of adverse reactions or even reaction to skin testing should not discourage the use of necessary immunizations. Also, based on these results, it seems that the use of skin testing to assess tetanus toxoid response is unfounded, because response to skin testing is inconclusive.

Maryann A. Green, Pharm.D. Student, Drug Information Service

cc: Carol M. Lane, Pharm.D., Director, Drug Information Service

1.   Jacobs RL, Lowe RS, Lanier BQ. Adverse reactions to tetanus toxoid. *JAMA* 1982;247:40-2.

Alan Harris, Pharmacist   October 3, 1993
Main Street Pharmacy
1234 Main Street
Barett, WA 97765

Dear Alan:

In follow-up to our telephone conversation on October 1, 1993, I have copied for your review two articles which support the use of cyclical etidronate for the treatment of osteoporosis in postmenopausal women.[1,2] Although the treatment protocol varies slightly between the Danish study[1] and the multicenter U.S. study[2], both studies demonstrated that in women with established postmenopausal osteoporosis (one to four vertebral fractures and radiographic evidence of vertebral osteopenia), etidronate 400 mg per day for 14 days repeated every three months, for two[2] or three[1] years, resulted in a significant increase in vertebral mineral content, and a significant decrease in the rate of new vertebral fractures. Calcium supplementation was appropriate during the weeks the patient was not taking etidronate, but the two agents could not be given together out of concern that calcium (including that in dairy products) would interfere with etidronate absorption, which is recognized as poor (1-9% of administered dose).[2] Etidronate was well tolerated in both trials.[1,2] Side effects included nausea (5-6%) and diarrhea (79%). For a subgroup of patients (n=55) who underwent bone biopsy studies, no osteomalacia was evident in any pretreatment biopsy sample; no mineralization defect was seen in any post-treatment sample.[2]

Although the use of etidronate for the treatment of osteoporosis falls outside the current product labeling, the available clinical evidence supports consideration of etidronate for women who closely match the populations studied in the trials described. Unfortunately, brief reports of these findings have found their way into the lay press, but the important supporting descriptions of which patients might benefit from treatment with etidronate have often been lost in the presentation. Consumers who perceive themselves to be at risk for osteoporosis and are seeking "prophylaxis" clearly fall outside the group who might benefit.

I hope the etidronate trials will help you discuss this promising new treatment of osteoporosis with physicians and patients. Please feel free to call on us if we may be of further assistance.

Katie L. Jones, Pharm.D., Drug Information Services   Enclosures (2)

References

1. Storm T, Thamborg G, Steiniche T, Genant HK, Sorensen OH. Effect of intermittent cyclical etidronate therapy on bone mass and fracture rate in women with postmenopausal osteoporosis. *N Engl J Med* 1990;322:1265-71.
2. Watts NB, Harris ST, Genant HK, et al. Intermittent cyclical etidronate treatment of postmenopausal osteoporosis. *N Engl J Med* 1990;323:73-9.

Index